UNIMACY
LOVE AND INTIMACY
THAT LASTS

LARA ANDERSON

BALBOA.
PRESS

A DIVISION OF HAY HOUSE

Balboa Press books may be ordered through
booksellers or by contacting:

Balboa Press
A Division of Hay House
1663 Liberty Drive
Bloomington, IN 47403
www.balboapress.com
1 (877) 407-4847

Because of the dynamic nature of the Internet, any web addresses or
links contained in this book may have changed since publication and
may no longer be valid. The views expressed in this work are solely those
of the author and do not necessarily reflect the views of the publisher,
and the publisher hereby disclaims any responsibility for them.

The author of this book does not dispense medical advice or
prescribe the use of any technique as a form of treatment for physical,
emotional, or medical problems without the advice of a physician,
either directly or indirectly. The intent of the author is only to offer
information of a general nature to help you in your quest for emotional
and spiritual well-being. In the event you use any of the information
in this book for yourself, which is your constitutional right, the author
and the publisher assume no responsibility for your actions.

Any people depicted in stock imagery provided by Thinkstock are
models, and such images are being used for illustrative purposes only.
Certain stock imagery © Thinkstock.

Print information available on the last page.

ISBN: 978-1-5043-7907-6 (sc)
ISBN: 978-1-5043-7908-3 (e)

Balboa Press rev. date: 05/10/2017

Love, care and acceptance when embraced bodily open a new understanding of sexuality that needs to be taught to all generations of men and women now more than ever.

This book is dedicated to all the men and women who do not possess physical perfection but the perfection of the heart.

Human sexuality is a beautiful language through which we can express love. When one person is touching another they bring the loved one into an ocean of happy feelings. When these feelings are felt deeply in both partners their love becomes energy for the universe. Yet, we need to create this language of love, take care of its beautiful sound and be grateful for its blessing to be able to speak and listen to it.

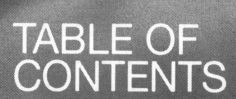

TABLE OF CONTENTS

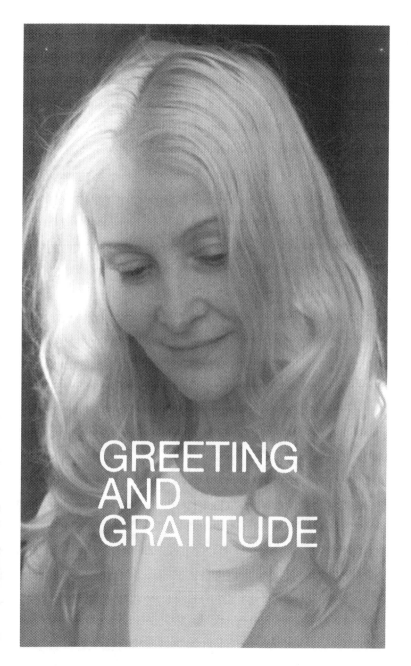

GREETING
AND
GRATITUDE

Welcome!

You have opened this book.

It means that you have questions about your sexual happiness. Yet, it does not mean that something is wrong with your sexual life. This book is not like many other guides about how to improve certain skills. This book does not belong to the series so popular these days saying: "Do as I do and you will achieve the same results." This book is not about results because there are no results in sexuality. Most people do not know how to live in love every minute and how to express this feeling via the body without fear, complexes, confusion and embarrassment. But everyone understands that physical love is the foundation for lasting affection, that a deep emotional and erotic experience of intimacy is the supreme embodiment of love between a man and a woman.

This book can totally change your life. It can create a revolution in your mind and open you up to a rich palette of physical sensations. These sensations are available to you. You can offer these sensations to yourself and to the body of your lover as long as you live on this earth. What is most interesting, your body knows these sensations but does not allow itself to experience them. This book presents a system that will help you remove all the obstacles for giving and receiving love fully and creatively. People of different nationalities and different faiths come to see me. Many of them read great books, meditate, do yoga and listen to spiritual teachers... Many of them are balanced and happy. Yet when it comes to sexuality they are completely lost. They can not make this part of their lives as satisfactory as other parts. Like nowhere else, in sexuality it is not enough to understand with your mind. In fact here the physical interaction with another body means everything. That's why only practical learning can help you create sexual happiness, and thereby love, every day. This book presents only the theoretical part of my teaching. The real life support you will get from my practical courses and workshops. Though to engage in the practice you first need to obtain a new understanding of the nature and importance of sexuality in human life, as well as become acquainted with the main principles of my system.

My system is aimed at heterosexual couples because this is the range of my experience. However, gay people may benefit from Unimacy too.

I would like to dedicate this book to my friend Elena Magazova who inspired me to write this book. I would also like to thank Monica Andersson and Graham Perry for their countless hours spent reading this work, and for their suggestions and corrections. I would also like to express my deepest gratitude to my daughter Snezhana Kuzmina, the art director of this project. Finally, I am also very grateful to the photographers of the images used in this book: Daniel Santella (the cover image, page 79), Chuttersnap (page XV), Christopher Campbell (page 1), Alvin Mahmudov (page 17), Freestocks.org (page 43), Elisabeth Tsung (page 111) and Valeria Boltneva (page 115).

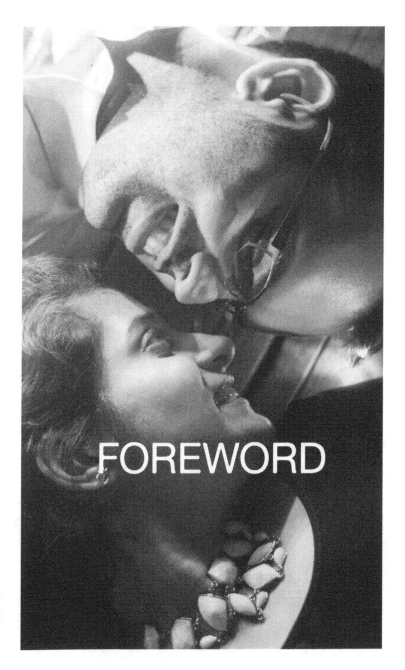

FOREWORD

The sexual relationship is the most difficult area of human life and the most delicate and painful subject for many couples.

"Maybe we should try to have sex again?" the woman asked the man. He paused and seemed not to hear the question. The woman touched the man's arm. He turned his head toward her. She repeated: "Maybe we should try to have sex?" He looked away to the sea. "Why do you suddenly think that?" the man asked after a long pause. "It would bring us closer," the woman replied with despair in her voice. The man did not know what to say. They stood for a long time on the deck in silence. Finally the man put his arm around the woman's shoulders and said, "You are very dear to me, I love you very much. You are the best wife in the world. Come on." The man took the woman into the cabin. They went to bed, as usual in their pyjamas. The man immediately fell asleep. The woman stared out into the darkness as her eyes were welling up with tears.

We all want to be intimate with the person who is dear to us...

"Please can you help me? I am a married man 35 years of age.

I have been married for 6 years however the sexual relationship with my wife has been quite poor. This has created such a tremendous strain in our relationship that my wife has started to consider separation.

The issues I have are:

1. *Inability to ejaculate during intercourse. I am able to ejaculate when I masturbate but not able to do so during intercourse.*

2. *Inconsistent penis erection. Sometimes I manage to have a strong erection but other times I am unable to do so. I take medical stimulants like Viagra to overcome this issue but I still lack in confidence.*

3. *I am not able to arouse my wife. She feels my techniques are very crude and do not make her feel aroused. We have an extremely low frequency of intercourse due to above issues which now has an impact on all aspects of our lives. I want to save my relationship."*

Sexuality is a very important part of everyone's life and it affects us in the most powerful way. Being sexually attractive is everyone's deep and fundamental desire. It gives us tremendous confidence, power, inspiration, energy and a sense of well-being.

We all believe that we deserve intimacy.

This is true; we are all born sexual beings and human beings!

We also believe we know how to be intimate and that we have a lot to offer our lovers. This is not always true. We agree that making love confirms and maintains our bond with our partners. We know that sexual happiness helps the relationship; it provides stability and security. We want stable relationships as it gives us companionship, better health, more confidence and many other joys. Deep down we want to make love at any age and after many years of marriage. However, **most of us do not know what making love is or how to make love instead of 'having sex'.** Because of this a lot of men and women go through love dramas, once or several times in life. The truth is that everyone feels wonderful in the beginning of a new intimate relationship! And everyone feels awful when the intimate life starts to become problematic.

Unfortunately most intimate relationships start to have problems after a time. Why? Because the body gets older and the natural physiological desire based on hormone production - which, by the way, has nothing to do with love - ceases. Because we get used to our long term partner and the initial triggers, like appearance, novelty and sexual longing for our partner, do not work any more. Because the sexual techniques we used for years become a boring routine. Because our bodies can no longer perform the physical actions aimed to stimulate sexual arousal that we performed when we were younger. However, the main reasons for our problems with sex are a limited understanding of sexuality and an undeveloped skill when it comes to lovemaking.

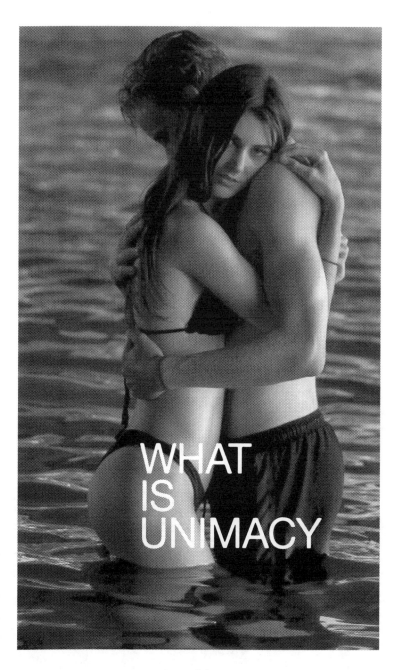

WHAT
IS
UNIMACY

What Is Intimacy?

Most people do not realise just how much intimacy depends on their **physical body**, on how they perceive it, how they treat it and how they interact with another physical body. Most people would not agree with the above statement. But be honest with yourself. When you think about intimacy, what pictures come to your mind first? I am sure that your thoughts are around your own and your lover's body. You think about holding hands, kisses, hugs and sex, don't you? You would not feel intimate with someone who is physically unattractive to you. You would not want to touch that person's body. On the other hand you would consider being in love with a person who's body creates in your mind a desire to touch it. Also, if you are attracted to someone you might worry about your own physical body. Will your body be attractive to that person? Will this person want to touch you? Intimacy is not present if you are not able to touch the body of your loved one. Intimacy is dead if you do not feel a desire to touch your partner's body.

Unfortunately the fact that the physical body is the main source of attraction, joy and worry, has a very strong impact on the relationship. If your physical body does not feel comfortable, is not aroused enough, is hurt, or doesn't reach orgasm, you might conclude that your partner is not good for you. You might end a relationship with a person who could really be your true soul mate and a wonderful partner in all other aspects of your life. How your physical body interacts with the body of your partner can maintain or destroy the relationship.

"*Dear Lara,*

My girlfriend and I love each other very much and we do want to have a long lasting relationship; unfortunately sex does not work. I am too fast and like fire I get excited too quickly. She does not feel sexual desire (in general). In fact in the last few months we have been able to do it only a few times. We have tried to massage each other, loving touch, yoni massage etc. etc. but it doesn't work and I cannot light my girlfriend's fire for love making. We are both very upset and discouraged. We want to be happy together, we want to laugh and have fun and fulfil each other lives but this sex thing is complicating everything....!!!!"

"*Dear Lara,*

My name is Kate. I am in a relationship where I have encountered sexual problems for the first time in my life. The main issue is that my boyfriend is 'really big' and if I am not wet enough, it really hurts. Because of this it is even hard for me to stay wet. I do not feel as aroused anymore as I once did. I do not feel sexual anymore and it is affecting our ability as a couple to 'go all out'. I want once again to feel vibrant and aroused. Another issue is that I can't do all the positions anymore that I once did because it hurts... I have read about this and I know I need to be really wet and hot. But I do not feel hot or very sexual at the moment... I have lost something. I used to be really into tantra, kama sutra, exploring my sexuality and at the moment I feel really bad in bed something I never thought I would be. I want to save what little is left of my sexuality... I feel a bit dead inside.

Most men and women are convinced that they can do nothing to repair a sexual relationship, that sexual happiness should exist by itself like the sunrise exists in the nature. Most men and women are looking for an uncontrolled and spontaneous rise of sexual energy (arousal) in their bodies so they feel drawn to people who can make their bodies feel this way. Because of this they can make mistakes in choosing the right partner for themselves.

Is it possible to firstly, control your sexual desire and direct it towards the person who can be a good partner for life, and secondly, develop sexual happiness? Yes, I am sure of this. It is possible to get a new insight into your sexual happiness. There are a lot of things men and women have to consider and think about when confronted with sexual problems. Life is a constant teacher and what we had in the past is only partially relevant to our present. Life is given to us to change, to grow and to learn new things, including when it comes to our physical body and the body of our partner.

Even so, the emotional exchange is the key to sexual happiness.

The Downside Of The Sexual Revolution

More than forty years ago the world was shaken by the sexual revolution. Women became sexually expressive and more active. They were introduced to the idea of having 'GO' – Great Orgasms and they started to strive for that. However, not every kind of orgasm - not even the most powerful one - creates between two sexual partners an experience of deep connection, intimacy and devotion. There is also proof that having many orgasms and having them often might even cause health problems. In the past men were mostly searching purely for sexual and physical gratification. Today women also want that. Both men and women have started to have more sexual partners. Yet they have to consider the dangers to their health and well-being that come with sex through infections or activation of certain bacteria.

The sexual revolution proclaimed sexual freedom. Unfortunately this freedom did not help many men and women find happiness in their relationships. Rather the opposite: it brought higher expectations of orgasmic pleasure and created more fear, complexes and unhappiness in people's sex lives and relationships.

Sexual desire is instant and very powerful but **sexual desire does not mean intimacy.** In my opinion the sexual revolution was a proclamation of freedom for the simple sexual instinct. Today we live in a world that advertises sexual pleasure literally 24/7. The huge market for sexual services, sex toys, pornography and even mainstream sexual education, develops in men and women a desire for pure physical sexual gratification instead of encouraging them to develop deeper love. All of this disconnects the feeling of love from sexual pleasure in people's minds. Because of this many men and women have given up on their sexual happiness, especially those who are married or living in a long term relationship. Often a couple's sex life becomes a boring routine focused on reaching climax or one partner demands from the other his or her physical pleasure. The absence of a happy sex life inevitably creates a huge distance between partners. Longing for love brings people together yet sex often separates them. Why? Uncontrollable sexual desire, passion, physical actions towards reaching orgasm can all be demanding, stressful, exhausting and often even painful for our physical body, as well as impact on our emotional state. In the sexual act there are two people involved which means both will struggle if the sex life is not satisfactory for one of them.

Why We Need Sexual Evolution

We need freedom **from instinct.** We need to learn how to develop as loving sexual beings, how to evolve in our relationships towards the feeling I call 'physical love'. The best way to experience sexual pleasure is to have the same regular sex partner and develop with him or her a fulfilling and healthy sexual relationship.

Intimacy between partners will be more likely to survive if the sex life becomes a more regular, nurturing practice with no expectations, no goal and therefore no disappointment. Acceptance, care, physical and emotional balance are the keys to sexual happiness. Physical love is not just sex, it is much more! The same partners can make love every day for the rest of their lives if making love is a soulful process that creates the necessary feelings of bonding and connection. This more intimate kind of sex will give a man and a woman extraordinary strength and vitality. They will reach an incredibly deep sense of oneness with each other. They will feel as though they stand on this earth not on two feet, but on four ... no, on thousands of feet.

Why I Have Written This Book

During my 20 years of practice as a holistic sex therapist I have met many women and men who lost interest in sex or were even scared of sex. Even the ones that considered sex to be a good thing had sexual experiences that were dull and boring or dramatic, even traumatic. Often my clients could not see what was positive about sex. They were blaming themselves or their partners and this obviously badly impacted their relationships. They did not know how to make love in any other way than the way most men and women do, the way it is presented by mainstream sex educators and the wider media. They did not know how to develop a conscious and respectful attitude towards their own body and the body of their partners. The body has limitations, but even so it can be a source of endless joy and energy when its needs are taken care of with the intention of balancing the body rather than arousing it more and more.

In a global perspective I have met just a tiny drop in the ocean of the men and women who are sexually confused or embarrassed or who feel fear and emotional pain when it comes to sex.

Caring for and cultivating one's sexual activity is not a new idea. Even so that knowledge was never presented to a wider public in any society. We live in the 21st century but talking about sex, teaching sex and sexual healing for a good sex life is still taboo and a very difficult task. It is difficult because throughout the time of human civilisation we have not created the right culture for sex. We have not created the right sex education to teach boys to respect female bodies and to teach girls to help boys to deal with their sexual instinct. We have not created institutions that prepare educators and therapists to teach men and women how to physically love each other. Universities educate psychiatrists and sexual therapists, often people who haven't mastered sexual desire themselves. Freud, Jung and others did write about the influence of sexual desire on people's psychology but they did not offer answers to the question of how to deal with this desire. Most importantly, none of them viewed sex as an expression of love and care for another person, nor suggested any physical techniques (touches) for such an expression. Yet, it is touch and touch alone that creates emotion and thereby affects our psychology.

In this book I share my personal view on sexuality as a woman who has been sexually close to many men in my personal and professional life as a tantric teacher. My knowledge is based on my many years of practical exploration of the difficulties experienced by those I have worked with and spent time with.

I have been researching not so much the subject of seduction so popular these days, instead my genuine desire has been to find an answer to the question of how to maintain sexual happiness with the same partner during one's whole life. In this book I will describe the main principles and ideas I have discovered and that I invite you to incorporate into your life if you want to create a long lasting relationship as opposed to merely wanting to 'pick up' someone.

Sexuality is a subject that has been researched for generations. However, in many ways sexuality is an individual and subjective path. Also it belongs to our creative nature, to our hearts and our irrational minds. It is like the ability to sing beautifully. The most useful and correct knowledge that a man or a woman can find can only come from their own experiences. So it was for me too. My experiences are suggestions to others. Though I strongly believe in my teaching because I have seen the results of the advice I have given.

We live in a time where people are focused on achievements. And there is nothing wrong with that, nothing wrong with motivation and setting goals! However, intimacy is not a thing that can be created through power, hard work, right decision making or even by the long journey of self-improvement or by embracing spirituality. Intimacy is a fragile and mystical experience. It can only be approached when the ego is dropped, when wonder and gratitude are present.

What Is Unimacy?

My system is called Unimacy from the combination of the two English words 'union' and 'intimacy'. 'Union' for me represents the oneness that two partners feel when making love. 'Intimacy' means openness, truth, a sharing of problems and finding solutions together in life and in sex.

The aspirations that led me to creating this concept were:

- To feel loved.
- To improve health.
- To slow down ageing and extend life.
- To help men and women love each other.
- To help parents educate their children about sexual life.

I wanted my system to work in my own relationship. However I strongly believe that my system can help any couple at any stage of their sexual relationship, even when intimacy is completely absent in their life. Using my practical methods and system anyone can create beautiful sexual communication bringing both partners physical and emotional happiness. This will then open the way for them to communicate this knowledge to their children.

Why is Unimacy a system?

If we do something regularly it means that we have a system. By repeating the same actions over and over again what we create becomes a habit. Unimacy offers a practice to do this, which if done every day provides security in a relationship as it provides a sustainable love life. Every day partners touch each other, they express love and because of that they feel loved. The Unimacy system also helps partners express their love differently every time which prevents their sexual life from becoming routine and boring.

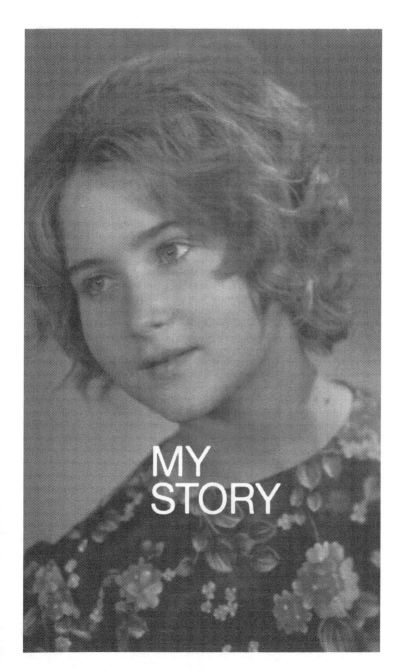

MY
STORY

I was seventeen years old when I had my first sexual intercourse. It happened with a man I was in love with. We had known each other for more than two years. It seemed as if we were already great lovers. We could spend hours stroking, kissing and hugging each other. We experienced warm pleasant waves of arousal in our genitals and told each other about it, yet we held back the desire for intercourse.

We were extremely happy without intercourse. Incredible admiration of each other's bodies was expressed by constant compliments, observation and touch. We did it everywhere: in the street, on buses, at the movies... When we were alone in the room we could slowly and gently stroke each other for hours, rediscovering again and again every curve and every hill of our bodies. We kissed each other's bellies, necks, legs, arms, faces... In the shower our hands slipped over each other's soapy skin like water... We touched each other so wonderfully and derived so much pleasure from each other!

Our rich world of physical love gradually became narrow and dull after intercourse started to become a part of our relationship. Very soon I started to dislike more and more our quick strip and brief activity under the blankets. Often I suffered pain caused by the rigid movements of my boyfriend's penis in my vagina. I tried to change his behaviour and to introduce him to my understanding of sex, which was slower and gentler, but he would not let me. We did not succeed in reviving the previous poetic touches. A year later we broke up.

As a young woman I started to explore my sexual feelings. I wanted to feel loved. I tried to understand my body more. I wanted always to enjoy sexual encounters with a man.

So in my youth I decided that I would make love like slow dancing. I believed that lovemaking should not consist of any pressure or excessive excitation. I decided always to initiate this dance myself. By doing this, I hoped to prevent my man from rushing. I did not want him to concentrate only on his own sensations and on bringing himself faster to ejaculation. I decided to teach my man how to touch me and help him to relax.

I got married when I was 21. The 10 years of marriage to my first husband was sexually a very happy time. He tragically died at 35. At his death I was left with two small children and have not had an easy life. Though having lovers has helped me a lot and I have shared a lot of pleasure with my partners.

So what was my unique skill as a lover that always made me happy as a woman and sexually attractive to the man I made love with? From an early age I had learnt these things:

- A motherly attitude to my own body and to the body of my partner.
- Everything was initiated by me.
- I never used any seductive elements.
- I learned to control the intensity of sexual arousal through the movements of my body and invited the man to follow my body.
- I always kept the attention on my partner not on myself.
- I was not focused on achieving an orgasm but on having a lot of sweet waves passing through my whole body.
- I always tried to help my partner to experience the same waves, thereby balancing his body sexually and avoiding ejaculation.

- I always nurtured my partner's body.
- I always refused to have sexual encounters with anyone trying to seduce me or wanting me to behave seductively.

I really initiated everything I wanted to do during sex. I did not wait for my lover to act upon my body. I have never used any seductive elements during lovemaking: my face always looked angelic with a warm soft smile, my body moved with beautiful innocent playfulness, I never moaned loudly or shouted. If I wanted to be 'wild' and drive myself and my partner to a higher state of arousal I still moved as if I was dancing. I maintained strong connection with my partner rather than focusing on rubbing my genitals against his body. Nurturing my partner in a motherly manner became more and more rewarding for me. Stroking, massaging and kissing him was for me expressing my sexuality in this caring, innocent and creative way. It tremendously enriched my own physical and emotional experience. I was happier when I saw my partner relaxed and smiling at me, following my movements. I did not like it at all when my lover got tense and wanted to bring himself or me to orgasm.

Though I have to admit that in the beginning with every man I felt that he wanted to dominate my body, more or less. I did understand that this male behaviour was based on his purely instinctive sexual desire for me. So I patiently brought the man into my world of romantic love and he gradually relaxed and gave up trying to force me into anything. Soon the man I made love with more and more enjoyed our soft and gentle lovemaking. I had total control over our lovemaking. I could make whatever movements I needed to bring my sexual energy to a comfortable level of intensity. It helped my man to keep his sexual energy at the same level as mine. Often my lover and I could make love for an hour or more and neither of us needed to finish with orgasm.

During my first sexual relationship I had already noticed that after having an orgasm, for a few days I had a very low energy. Sometimes the morning after lovemaking I could not go to the university. I never drank alcohol, I did not smoke, I did not go to bed late and my boyfriend and I mostly made love in the daytime. Still, the day after lovemaking I was absolutely exhausted. My head was heavy, often I felt nauseous and I started to avoid having an orgasm.

My life took me to different parts of Russia and then to England. I made a lot of friends. All of them would talk openly about their sexual experiences. My ideas of making love slowly and gently as well as the idea of avoiding orgasm were appreciated and absorbed into the lives of many of my friends.

I was in my late thirties when I started my professional sexual therapy practice. Ideas from Taoism, Tantra, medicine, psychology and even quantum physics have shaped my way of working. Also, my professional and personal experiences have provided me with a deep insight into the dynamics of sexual relationships and helped me to understand the changes in sexual behaviour that come with age.

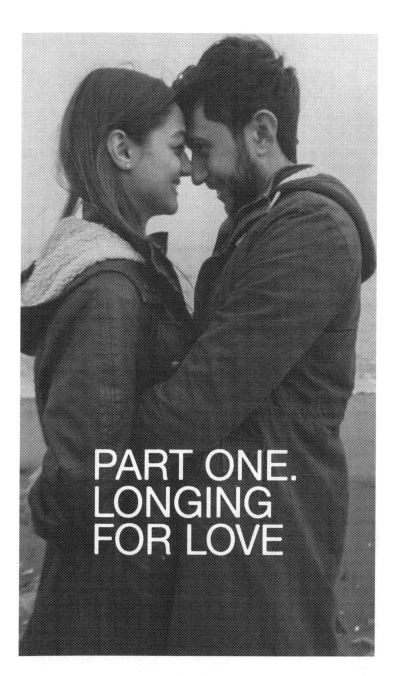

PART ONE.
LONGING
FOR LOVE

What I Have Heard From Men

A man, 56 years old: "We have been married for 22 years, have three wonderful daughters. I love my wife dearly. Our sex life used to be great! But over the last years my wife no longer gets as excited about sex as before. I have tried everything: made a nice dinner, taken her to a wonderful restaurant, given presents. Before we usually played a lot of erotic games, used toys and watched erotic films. Now she does not want any of that. She says: "I want soul connection. I cannot do that physical stuff anymore..." I do not understand her words..."

Me: "Your wife is getting older. Her body is not having the same instinctual sex drive as when she was younger. Maybe it is time to change your sexual practice from exciting and thrilling into something more loving, tactile, relaxing and nurturing? I can teach you that."

The man: "I know what you mean. But I need sex. I am full of energy. I am only 56 and my body needs sex every day. Now we have sex only 3-4 times a week. My wife is always tired. I cannot live like this."

Me: "If you develop a nurturing practice you will feel more sexually balanced..."

The man: "I understand what you mean. But I do not want to lose my desire for passion. I love it! I feel bored and I don't get excited from my wife massaging me. I love active sex. I have a good business and my children are almost grown up. I need a sexy woman!"

Me: "Do you mean that it is possible that you will leave your wife?"

The man: "I came here to learn new tips on how to make my wife sexy again!"

That man left me disappointed. He never called again. I thought with sadness of his wife.

Another man, 34 years old: "I want to stop my addiction to porn. I feel bad when I sit every evening in my study, watch porn and masturbate. I love my wife but I want her to do what women do in porn. I feel awful doing this. We are a wonderful family. We have two boys. I don't know how to stop my desire for porn. I am afraid of losing my wife because she isn't happy to do what I ask her to do."

Me: "What will you tell your two sons about sex when they get older? Would you teach them to treat women the same way you treat your wife?"

The man: "Exactly! I do not want them to be like me! I want them to be happy!"

Me: "I can teach you how to love your wife differently."

Two months later, the same man: "Thank you! My wife is much happier now. I am not watching porn at all! We do swap massages every day and so physically love (your expression!) constantly. We feel that we are so much in love! I can teach these massages to my sons when they are old enough!"

A man, 27: "I love my partner but I like to have other lovers. When we have sex she is very needy. She is getting so emotional, she is crying. She is begging me. I feel really uncomfortable. I look around and see strong women and I like them. My partner is very strong in other aspects of life. Only in sex she is weak and begging me to love her. It is very off-putting."

Me: "It seems like your partner wants you to love her in a deeper way. It means her body needs more loving touches from you not just sex. I can teach you that."

One month later, this same man: "My partner is very happy when I do to her what you taught me. Yet I still want to have sex with other women. Why?"

Me: "Does your partner give the same massages to you?"

The man: "No. I asked her but she doesn't seem to think that she needs to do the same to my body."

Me: "Ask her to talk to me."

The man: "I did. She does not want to..."

I felt for this man. He was making an effort, but his partner wasn't.

A man, 54: "We are happily married. Two grow-up daughters. My wife is a school teacher and works hard... We have not had sex for 20 odd years, since our second daughter was conceived. I always ejaculated very soon, sometimes even before entering her vagina... I feel I have wasted my life and did not love my wife properly. I want to change it. I want to love her physically. But I am scared..."

I worked with this man. After a few meetings with me he obtained a wonderful control of his arousal and ejaculation. However, sadly, he could not share this with his wife. She was not interested in sex any more.

A man, 38: "My wife is a very beautiful woman. She is also a very good business woman, she runs a big company. We have three small children. I cannot satisfy her. She does not like me to massage her, stroke or kiss her. She wants me to be very dominating, forcing her, almost like raping. I cannot do that. We often go to swing parties. I cannot have sex with other women but my wife loves to have sex with a lot of men. I watch her doing this... I feel very unhappy... I love her so much."

I worked with this couple in one long session. The man had tears in his eyes when his wife looked into his eyes and held his penis in her hand. He said that she never did this before. They left my studio with happy faces, but I was not sure that his wife would stop looking for sexual thrills.

What I Have Heard From Women

A woman, 34: "I feel I cannot pretend any more that I am happy with our sex life. My husband is a wonderful man and we have two kids. Even so I don't want to have sex with him because it's always the same; he enters me painfully and ejaculates within two minutes."

After a few sessions during two months this woman wrote to me: "Me and my husband are now on a magical journey of physical love that I feel will never end."

A woman, 39: "We have been married for three years. My husband is 42. We are real soul mates! We care a lot about each other. Even so I am still a virgin. We both want a proper family. We want a child. But we do not know how to start having sex. My husband seems very nervous when I try to initiate sex..."

I worked with this couple for three hours and the next day I received an email from the wife: "Yesterday you helped us to bond at a level we have missed for three years of our married life... I am still in shock as to how much we covered with you and the levels we reached. In so many ways I want to shed a tear of joy but I'm holding back. Anything is possible if you just love the other person... I am on cloud nine!" During the session I had understood that this woman's husband was very tired, he was working hard and was often away. I suggested to her that she initiate physical contact herself by giving loving massages to her husband. He was very happy with that. I contacted the woman a few weeks later and she wrote to me: "We are making progress, it's slow but we are getting there. I did not feel comfortable initiating touch. I've always wanted the man to take charge. It was an awkward thing for me to do..."

I recommended her to continue trying what I had already suggested and contacted her again after a few weeks. It seemed like they still did not achieve physical closeness. I can only say that anyone can have what they want if they really want it. I was there to help them take further steps towards their happiness if they so desired.

A woman, 31: "My partner and I are running three pubs. We have 30 employees. We work from 7am until 12 pm. Both of us are very tired. I feel that our love is fading and I do not feel like a woman anymore. We hardly make love anymore... maybe once a month now and my partner ejaculates quickly. There is no passion, no energy... I feel very sad."

This couple was easy to teach. Both of them realised under my guidance that they do not need to wait for passion. Learning techniques on how to relax each other, how to give loving massages and taking on board my advice to connect through penetration every day even for five minutes they found a deeper love. They wrote to me after three weeks saying that they now had much more energy, they were as happy as they had been in the beginning of the relationship and they planned for lovemaking 2-3 hours on Mondays, when the pubs were closed.

A woman, 22: "My boyfriend and I have known each other for four years. I want to make love to him but I'm always so tense and nervous... We started to have sex two years ago. During this time we have separated a few times. All because of sex. He gets irritated because I do not enjoy sex and just wait until he ejaculates. He wanted to leave me but we got back together because we have so much in common and are very happy in many other ways. We are both creative artists."

This young woman, like many young women, was not able to relax. Her boyfriend, like many young men, was physically forceful. During the session with me they learned a lot of loving nurturing techniques and experienced very loving and gentle intercourse. The girl contacted me after a few months with gratitude confirming that they have developed a very loving sexual relationship.

A woman, 57: "I love to be physical with my husband. I love it when he hugs me, strokes or kisses me, but he always worries about his erection. He does not have a good erection any more. I said to him: "I don't need your erection." I love to be intimate without penetration. I give him oral. Even so he asks me to masturbate his penis a lot and gets angry if he cannot come. When I cannot make him come he doesn't want to hug and kiss me..."

This couple visited me for a four hour session. They enjoyed my teaching a lot though the husband was very nervous all the time because he did not have a good erection. I recommended him to do the solo training I teach in my course for men and which has helped a lot of my clients. I also recommended his wife to give him more loving massages. A month later his wife wrote to me that she gives her husband massages but he has not changed, he still wants to ejaculate and gets angry if he cannot. My comment to this situation is that anyone can make their sexual relationship happy if they want to and if they take steps towards the happiness of their partner. This husband did not think about his wife.

Why People Are Unhappy Sexually

Through my life and work I have realised that many people do not understand the meaning of sex as being bonding, connection and care. Today a lot of men and women fear sexual relationships the same way people fear public speaking. They see sex as a performance and feel it is their responsibility to impress. Men and women worry that they will not be able to meet their partner's expectations in sex, whatever they see sex to be. However few people think about sex as love, care, acceptance and gentleness.

Men fear sexual relationships because they perceive their sexual desire and physiological functioning as very difficult to manage. Women fear sex because they feel that they are not sexually attractive enough. Often they experience physical discomfort in the vagina and emotional vulnerability.

Another reason why people are not happy sexually is that their attitude to sex is about 'consuming'.

What do we mostly hear from men and women?

1. "This girl is gorgeous! I would like to spend a night with her!
   or
2. "My boyfriend is so passionate! He gives me wonderful orgasms!"
   Not that often do we hear:
3. "I am very gentle with my girlfriend's body. I listen to her every breath and ask if she is comfortable with everything I do to her body."
   or
4. "My boyfriend is working hard. When he comes home I want him to relax and rest. I give him a

slow and gentle massage, kiss him all over and
make love to him slowly and gently. I want him to
feel loved by me."

Do you believe that your partner has the thoughts stated in
number 3 and 4 above? Do you often have similar thoughts
yourself?

There are two groups of men and women: those who
think that they do not know how to physically love and
those who believe that they do know how to physically
love. In most cases men and women from both groups
differ only in one thing: The ones in the first group don't
take physical action because they feel scared and nervous
about approaching a potential sexual partner. The ones
in the second group do act physically, which means they
simply go and have sex.

But let's have a closer look at these two groups in
relation to sexual fulfilment.

The first group of people think that they lack sexual
confidence because they haven't had enough sexual
experiences and because they have sexually unattractive
bodies. However, these men and women have a greater
chance of finding happiness and contentment in their
sexual relationships than the men and women from the
other group.

The bodies and minds of shy and less confident lovers
are not so prone to high expectations and an addiction to
'hot' pleasure. They are 'pure' on a biochemical level as
they have not developed an addiction to high arousal and
orgasm. These men and women haven't experienced a
sense of routine and habituation which means they do
not have bitterness or other negative emotions connected
with sex. Men and women from this group are able to care

more about their partners than about themselves and feel grateful for received love. They truly want to be lovable and loving and this is the secret to a happy relationship. But it only works when the caring attitude is mutual.

The second group of people are those who think they are sexually attractive, that they are 'great lovers' and always have great sex. These men and women follow mainstream beliefs about sex and about what sexual attraction is, who it means to be a great lover and what great sex is. Eventually most of these individuals will start to experience the downside consequences of their beliefs which I will describe further later in this book.

We live in a world of achievements. We have started to see relationships as part of the package together with other material values. This means however that if you haven't achieved a lot you do not deserve love. Love these days is associated with physical perfection as well as high professional achievements.

A lot of self-help speakers are right in that you have to strive for more in life and expect more of yourself. But when it comes to relationships this attitude is harmful and brings with it a sense of constant evaluation of your partner and yourself. This is powerfully reflected in sex and then in your relationships. Sexual relationships turn into a competition instead of becoming a home, a place to relax, to feel accepted and loved.

The reason for all this suffering is the fact that most people do not love their own bodies. They are not happy with their bodies as they constantly compare themselves with mainstream sex symbols. They don't know their bodies in their loving aspect and they don't understand that their sexual happiness comes from within, as does everything else in a person's life.

Without love, respect, care and management of our own sexuality we cannot be loving physically towards others. We will just be consumers of bodies and energies, including our own body and energy.

When we feel a physical desire for sex and don't satisfy it we can feel frustrated, irritable and nervous. Sexual tension can hinder our concentration on other things and even make us unable to do anything but think about sex. This is more common in men than in women.

We also need to love and feel loved, to have a long lasting loving relationship. Sadly the physiological need for sex and the desire for intimate connection do not always appear together in the human mind.

The instinctual desire to have sex comes upon us by itself without us having to do anything. It comes and goes chaotically and uncontrollably. In different bodies it has a different frequency and intensity of arousal. A feeling of intense sexual desire, the physical arousal called 'chemistry' or 'falling in love', often does not represent a desire for intimacy. Many men and women after a while feel less interest and passion for their regular partners when they feel diminished arousal in their bodies. The lack of passion (the uncontrollable sexual desire called libido) gives rise to a sense of insecurity and uncertainty. It creates worries in us about losing our partner and reduces our sense of confidence and well-being. This creates tension between partners, a sense of disconnection, feelings of jealousy, arguments and so on.

But the truth is, sexual desire satisfied via passionate sex and orgasm which most men and women consider to be good sex, at least for some time, does not create lasting sexual happiness. On the contrary, it is illusory and creates unhappiness as soon as the passion gets less intense and orgasm is not achieved.

Everyone comes into a relationship with the feeling that he or she will lead a sexually happy life. Though the passion often dies within 2-3 years and most partners cease to make love after 10 years of marriage. Finding the solution in a new sexual partner does not guarantee that this new relationship will not end in the same way. Nor does spicing up the sex life with games, toys or stimulating images help the relationship to survive. These tools and tricks do not create a sense of intimacy and love, they only stimulate arousal.

Men and women do not know that the physical capacity for arousal based on hormone production is very limited and starts to reduce from the age of 23 in both men and women. At 23 already! Add to that the fact that our sense of sexual desire towards our partner is reduced with time as a result of habituation.

We ought to treat sexuality with more respect and give it more importance than we do food. When we lose the desire to be physically close to our partner, we lose our partner. This is much more painful than when we eat badly. We need to **see sexuality as part of the feeling of love. And this feeling needs to be developed with creativity**. Anything that we allow to evolve by itself without our care, attention and awareness comes back to us as disappointment. So far most men and women do not care about developing the feeling of love. They are looking for more of a physical or visual stimulus to create physical arousal in their body, to build this up and then release it through physiological orgasm. There is no sense of intimacy in this process.

Everyone Longing For Love Can Create Love

You create love in the same way you create anything in life. **You need to focus on it and you need to focus on it consistently.**

The same way you focus on your work to get better at it and be promoted you need to know what is your focus in physical love.

What are the elements you need to develop and improve in order to maintain love?

Sexuality is viewed by a lot of people, including medical professionals and spiritual teachers, as something purely personal related to self-pleasuring.

Yes, sexual happiness comes from within as everything else in a person's life comes from within, but this is not the same as self-pleasuring.

In a sexual act with someone else you are not the only person involved. There are two people present – your partner and you. Note that I say: "your partner and you" instead of "you and your partner". When I talk about happiness from within what I mean is loving and giving this body of yours as a gift to your partner. **The pleasure you get when making your partner happy creates sexual happiness within you.** Not reaching orgasm, not gaining you own sexual release, not feeling aroused. Your joy comes from touching and loving your partner's body for the sake of your partner's comfort and happiness. And your joy and pleasure comes from receiving your partner's physical love, touch, kisses and hugs in return.

The main focus of your sex life is your partner.

Do not worry that you may be left without pleasure if you give all your attention to your partner. This book is for partners to read together and to agree on sharing with each other in a mutual way. If your focus is your partner, then your partner's focus is you. It does not make sense to be together if this is not the case. A happy sex life and a happy relationship is not possible if each of the partners is focused on themselves.

How To Bring Unimacy Into Your Life

Read this book. Offer to your partner to read this book too. Discuss the things you have read. Help each other integrate the knowledge presented in this book on a theoretical level. Only after that can you start your physical practice. Only after embracing the beliefs and attitudes of this system can your physical expression of love become a steady agreed upon practice for both. And this will allow it to every time be a wonderful gift.

If you are single, obtain the knowledge first. Practice what will help you prepare for a relationship. Make up your mind about what type of partner you need. Look for this partner and when you meet the right person, read this book together with them. It does not make sense for you to have a partner that won't agree with the Unimacy path if that is the path you want to choose.

What is Physical Love within the Unimacy Teaching?

What is love? Love is the joy of being with that special person. Love means emotional and physical closeness with that person.

Then there is the word 'sex.' Maybe this word doesn't convey very well the wonderful experience people can create together expressing their love for each other. Maybe this word is too one-sided and limited, suggesting even if indirectly the act of copulation which any animal is capable of. Animals cannot make love however. Moreover, they can not create the erotic art of love. Maybe men and women would feel happier if they used the words 'making love' more often rather than the term 'having sex'?

I believe that the words 'making love' create a different state of mind, accompanied by completely different physical feelings and actions. If someone gently utters: "I want to make love with you," their physical behaviour will be more gentle and relaxed. They will pay more attention to the way they touch rather than focusing on achieving orgasm. However, even if the words "I want to make love with you" are pronounced many people do not know what to do physically unless they have intercourse.

The concept of 'Physical Love' is boundless. We will never stop loving physically if we expand our vision of physical closeness to include much more than the act of coitus. The longing for a merging of our bodies will never fade away if we learn to experience and circulate sexual energy in our bodies independently of external stimulus. Then the act of coitus will not be the one, the only or main important thing. If we cannot perform this act for some reason there is much more. Holding our partner in our arms, being aware of the body-to-body connection with our partner, of our emotional exchange, will give us an experience of deep intimacy and happiness.

It is clear to me that this vision of lovemaking is alien to most men and women. They cannot consider as sexual pleasure the act of holding each other. Read what my client, a 59 year old man, told me: "Every morning I do solo practice where I reach an orgasmic state in my body. It has nothing to do with my wife. This powerful flow of sexual energy for 10-15 minutes throughout my whole body recharges me for the day. I have time together with my wife every evening. Sometimes we have intercourse, sometimes not. Sometimes I have an erection, sometimes not. This does not affect the flow of sexual energy which creates connection and love between us. We lie still, we hold each other close, we are naked, we feel skin-to-skin contact, we feel our genitals pressing toward each other, we breathe in unison, we listen to our hearts beat... We are so happy! When I was young and did not know how to make love this way sex was definitely exhausting for me. I loved my wife but sometimes avoided physical contact with her as I felt no energy in my body."

Men and women need to gain knowledge about how the body, the sexual energy and the mind work. This will help them maintain a desire for making love consciously when there is not as much instinctual arousal in the body. Making love is similar to inspired singing. What makes us want to sing and learn how to sing well? Who needs that? We need it for ourselves. We create it ourselves if we want to. And if we do that, there is no end to the pleasure. It is like an ever-lasting orgasm.

The body of your partner can be like home, like a warm fire, an inspiration, a place to relax or become energised, a sweet elixir. Then you will always want to touch it, drink it in, immerse yourself in this world and merge your own world with your partner's world to fill both of you up with happiness. Union and intimacy are central to what is happening. If anyone in their physical lovemaking embarks on the path of conscious creation, the joy of connecting bodies will deepen every day and become a permanent and endless joy in life.

The keys to sexual happiness are **authenticity, genuine care and ultimate trust**. Also, human sexuality belongs to our creative human nature. We can all be sensual and sexual artists and as such maintain sexual attraction with the same partner for a lifetime if we develop our loving imagination.

The Five Senses

Physical love compounds feelings of love with sexual arousal and with our five senses. The body of a loved one creates in us a strong desire to touch him or her and it creates sexual arousal in our own body. We too want to be touched by the person we love and we want to be wanted by them sexually.

Physical love is not just touch. It includes all the five senses:

- Touch
- Sight
- Smell
- Taste
- Hearing

When we love someone we want:

- to touch the person,
- to look at him or her,
- to smell his or her smell,
- to taste his or her lips or other parts of their body,
- to hear their voice.

We also want to be physically loved the same way in return.

The Unimacy Aspirations

To expand sensuality within your own body.

Most people expect from sex powerful sensations purely in their genitals. It is as if the rest of the body is numb. Our brain wants these sensations and consequently it strongly directs our attention to the genitals. We need to re-educate our brain. We need to bring our attention to other parts of the body where our partner is touching us. Then we will not get bored and our partner will feel appreciated for the acts of love they direct towards our body. Then we will start to love our body more and also to love our partner more.

To help your partner expand the sensuality of their body.

The same usually happens when we touch our partner: we think only about their genitals. We think that we need to arouse him/her and for this reason stimulate their genitals. Instead we need to concentrate on creating feelings of love in our heart and focus on touching our partner's whole body radiating this feeling of love into it. We need to bring happy and cosy feelings into our partner's body. We allow our partner to respond to our touch with softness and relaxation. We gain softness and relaxation in our own body during our touching of the body of our partner. We create a sense of ease and comfort for our partner so that he or she can express their joy and happiness.

To develop better skills in romantic and arousing touch.

The sexuality given to us by nature is lacking in imagination and physical skills. Most people's imagination is based on the simple instinctual desire to get more and more aroused until finally reaching climax. Sexual tips and techniques help men and women obtain physical skills to arouse the body but they do not work on creating the sense of bonding and connection required to maintain good lovemaking long term.

This is why I have had in my practice a lot of broken-hearted men and women. Their partners left them for another lover, even though these clients told me that sex with their ex-partners was great.

This then makes you wonder what 'great sex' is. In the opinion of most people great sex is active stimulation to create arousal, passionate body movements and then orgasm. I doubt that if you say 'great sex' you think of slow gentle stroking and long kisses on the forehead or neck...

Romantic touch is different and too often hardly known amongst many men and women. Romantic touch creates romantic feelings. It is the type of touch reflected not in the part of our brain where we want more arousal and orgasm but in another part of our brain where we want to say: "I am so happy that I have you in my life! I love you so much! You are so wonderful!"

We all miss romance when it is not in our life. Romance stays an illusion until we learn to touch in ways that create the real feeling of romantic love. Romance is the dream of that special touch and the reality of experiencing it.

Usually romantic reality does not last long and too often returns back to being merely a romantic dream. This is because romantic touch needs to be supported by a strong feeling of adoration and care. When people have known each other for a long time the feeling of adoration fades. However, consciously strengthening it can make romantic reality last.

To expand the variety of romantic touch.

Romantic reality will last if your physical love consists of a variety of romantic touches. The physical body is vast. There are so many parts that we can touch with true loving feelings. We need to continually change our focus when we touch our partner's body. We need to create chains of touches which together encourage the flow of love. Your partner's body is like a land where you slowly travel and explore when you touch it with your hands, lips, skin...

To develop your ability to express Physical Love with all the Five Senses.

Arousal always brings our attention solely to the physical sensation. We need to learn to never stop enjoying our partner's taste, smell, appearance, the sound of their voice and breathing. Once more this comes down to our concentration and focus. If we widen our focus to experience our partner with all of our five senses and express our enjoyment of that experience, we make our partner feel special and so much happier. Our life is driven by pain and pleasure. The feeling of pleasure is our anchor. The pleasure of being loved completely, including the way we look, smell, sound, taste and feel to the touch creates a deep sense of being appreciated and therefore a deep sense of connection.

To develop your ability to receive and appreciate the Physical Love expressed to you trough your partner's Five Senses.

When our partner is touching us we need to consciously turn our five senses towards our partner. We enjoy their touch and express this enjoyment by looking at them with a smile and even adoration or we say nice words and make our voice sound beautiful to our partner's ears. We expand our sense of smell and breathe the smell of our partner into our lungs with a happy expression on our face... We synchronise our five senses with our partner's.

To replace instinctive sexual urges with conscious physical actions supported by Feelings of Care and Love.

When both partners expand their actions during sexual practice to the creation of a chain of romantic touches, their sexual instinct is naturally controlled by joyful sensations received through the five senses. The desire for higher arousal and the urge to climax disappear. Instead the bodies want to continue their magical exchange. This in turn supports trust and security as the exchange is based on care and love for the partner's body.

Creating A Unique Sexual Relationship

Can you imagine a sexual relationship based on mutual acceptance, kindness, tenderness, patience and tact? If your answer is yes, what do you have to worry about? No more need for worries!

To create a fulfilling, long lasting sexual relationship you only need to have two things in place:

- A mutual agreement with your partner to become conscious lovers in Unimacy, embracing union and intimacy in sex.
- Make love regularly.

How To Become A Good Lover.

- Set out on a journey of life-long exploration of your own and your partner's sexuality.
- Love yourself as a lover to someone else.

I will explain the above statements.

Your sexuality is constantly changing not only throughout your life but every day. It happens because the state of your body, the level of your sexual energy and the state of your mind are influenced by every day events. The same is true for your partner's sexuality. We cannot force our sexuality. We can only keep learning about it and create the right environment to express it.

Your sexuality is a gift to someone else. Your sexuality is an energy you can cultivate, accumulate and radiate to someone else. Your sexuality is the touch that makes your partner happy.

In the next part of this book I will introduce you to 17 principles, i.e. 17 Sex Beliefs that will allow you to consciously create a fulfilling sex life.

What Is Conscious Sex?

Instead of desiring passion and high arousal we can concentrate on respect and trust in relationship to our partner. We can consciously relax ourselves and establish a clear and calm state of mind. Our physical actions then create comfortable and cozy feelings in both bodies. When you are conscious in sex you stop worrying about performance and an end result in orgasm. You are confident because you are happy to listen to your partner's body and to your own, accept them, understand them, care for them and love them. You are learning what your bodies need today and you are giving that to your lover the same way your lover gives equal love and care to your body.

There is nothing unnatural or mind-blowing during conscious sex. There is a great sense of closeness and warmth. Everything is wonderful here and now, at each moment in time. Every touch is noticed and reciprocated. Boredom has no chance to appear as you and your partner are concentrating on each other.

Conscious sex is a sequence of conscious actions. It can be started any time and end any time. It never creates disappointment because it does not allow expectations. The only aim of conscious sex is to unite, to meet, to adore, to surrender, to wonder and to be grateful.

Conscious sex is a process and a process that gives energy. This process is never completed. This way there is no excessive physiological arousal. There is endless enjoyment of bodily contact between you and your partner. It is like a holiday. There is no effort required. During conscious sex your have an opportunity to observe your sensations and create more tactile feelings. In this process your sexual energy and the sexual energy of your partner are synchronised in waves of varying intensity. These waves do not form sharp peaks. Most of the time they stay at a comfortable level of intensity of arousal. You and your partner support each other in staying at that medium level while recognising the different states of each other's bodies.

Conscious sex can bring lovers into a valley of intense orgasmic waves ('valley orgasm') which eventually will raise the arousal to a higher level. Even though partners do not aim to reach a peak where they can release the build-up of sexual tension they can experience a wave of great intensity. This sensation can have a quality of completion. Yet, the energy is not lost. It was accumulated and assimilated by both partners into the whole body. During conscious sex you and your partner help each other raise the intensity of arousal gradually. You feed each other's sensations. Each one of you waits for the other on the way to a stronger wave. Each one of you can feel this wave simultaneously or almost at the same time.

Conscious sex creates a state of total happiness. If there is completion it is different from orgasm as understood by most people. The high intensity wave lasts longer and the way back down to a peaceful state of body and mind is also much longer. The whole process is slower and more gradual.

Conscious sex provides you with more life energy. The sense of love and happiness becomes apparent every minute of your life. This is true sexual happiness and it is possible at any age and after many years of marriage.

Learn To Control Your Sexual Desire

Our instinctual sex drive is uncontrollable like that of an animal. The more you allow this desire free reign the more it becomes wild, demanding and even more uncontrollable. The more you train the desire to serve your relationship the better it serves both you and your partner. This energy has to be channelled into a flame of sexual energy, supporting and supported by a feeling of love.

Our sexual desire can easily be kept under control by learning special techniques for directing sexual energy. There is always a risk of losing control at any moment.

From my own experience, every time I make love I feel in my body a desire to push towards higher arousal. But I know that as soon as I allow my arousal to increase I will have a desire for even more arousal. Then it will come to the point where I push it towards orgasm and lose connection with my partner. This means that I am no longer with him where he is. I will selfishly get my fix but the next day I will pay for it with low energy levels, a bad mood and an inability to think and work. It is true for me and for many others who have changed their sexual habits that high arousal and orgasm undermines or even destroys the energy and union with our partners.

In my practice I have had several couples with the following problem: the men complaining about not having an erection when wanting to have sex with their wives even though they loved them, but having an erection when by themselves.

I suggested that these couples make love every day for two weeks by connecting genitals for ten minutes with no other agenda. In just two weeks all men confirmed that they had much more energy in their bodies. All of the women who took my advice said the same thing. Both the men and the women also said that all the negative emotions they had had before were gone. The men stopped worrying about their erection and orgasm and men and women alike happily anticipated every chance to make love.

Deep down everyone just wants to live 'happily ever after' with the person he or she has chosen in their life.

Men and women should regularly express love sexually but keep instinctive sexual desire under control. Expressing love physically is an every day necessity to keep the feeling of love alive.

How To Create Sexual Happiness

There are four key elements to create sexual happiness:

The first: **Your beliefs.**

The second: **Your bodily skills.**

The third: **Communication with your partner.**

The fourth: **Romantic artistry.**

In this book I will lead you step-by-step through the first element of sexual mastery. The remaining three elements can only be partially presented in a book as a lot of learning and improvement need to be done through direct physical practice.

Sexual physical practice is like playing a musical instrument. You need constant practice even if you don't want to do too much at a time. Practice is life. You can create joy and love that last a lifetime if you actually make love every day. Practical suggestions from my system will greatly help you. You don't need to be well organised for lovemaking. My programs are easy to incorporate into your life.

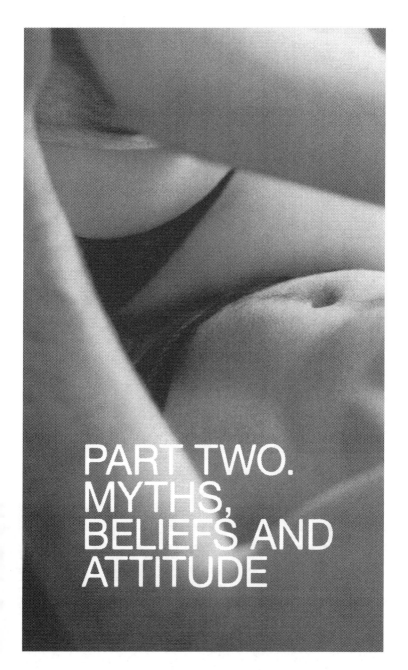

PART TWO.
MYTHS,
BELIEFS AND
ATTITUDE

Instinctual Sex And Peak Orgasm

Sex can be an act of fertilisation, sex can be intimacy and love, sex can be a sport, a game, a drug... You are the one who chooses what kind of sex you have.

Most people have only experienced instinctual sex and peak orgasm. Instinctual sex and peak orgasm are the only sexual behaviours considered to be normal by official institutions. Doctors, sex-therapists, psychiatrists, our educational system, churches and media give us advice on how to stimulate each other to achieve arousal and orgasm. This is in fact advice on how to reproduce but not on how to love each other physically. For many of these professionals and institutions the desire for sex (the so called libido) is considered to be a spontaneous impulse in the body that is stronger if our partner is likeable. If we do not feel a desire for sex in our body the same way we feel hunger it means, from this official viewpoint, that something is wrong with us. This is true from a limited biological perspective and this is what is officially established as normal sexual behaviour. Men and women have to have a regular drive for sex because for a male body it is important to fertilise, for a female body it is important to get pregnant and conceive. Most people believe in all that is said above.

The biological instinct switches on an attraction between men and women and this attraction is called falling in love. The relationship can develop into a loving and caring one but most people are engaged in sex simply because they enjoy the instinctual sexual impulse, the arousal in the body and the sense of euphoria at the moment of orgasm. No wonder that couples are not happy for long. They don't create a sense of bonding and connection but simply chase these sensations. Sexual harassment and rape are based on the same desire for sexual arousal in the body with no connection to love, affection, respect and care.

Physiological Orgasm: Yes Or No.

The idea that having sex means having a physiological orgasm is the mainstream belief concerning the aim of sexuality. This belief creates incredible limitations in our sex lives. It creates routine, boredom and tiredness. And there are a lot of other serious downsides and consequences that follow when we subscribe to this idea.

So what does this idea do to us?

- It creates demanding expectations in relation to our partner. If orgasm is not achieved we feel disappointed in our partner.
- It causes sexual problems. It is common for both men and women not to be able to achieve orgasm. A person might not have the energy for it and nevertheless try to bring themselves or their partner to orgasm, whether via intercourse, oral or manual stimulation. This causes physical fatigue, physical pain and emotional irritability and tension.
- When one partner is driving himself or herself to orgasm the other partner can feel that his or her body is being used and experience feelings of alienation and resentment.
- Persistent aspirations towards achieving orgasm can scare our partner and result in them trying to avoid sexual contact. This desire to avoid sex can extend to all physical contact - a hug,

a kiss, any type of touching including holding hands. The person might start to fear that even innocent touch will eventually lead to the initiation of sexual contact during which he or she has to provide an orgasm. Any contact can subconsciously be perceived as a danger in that it might involve a 'task' rather than pleasure. An orgasm exposes the internal organs to an excessive amount of stress. The fatigue that comes after orgasm indicates this loss of energy. Frequent loss of energy exhausts the body and mind and reduces the ability and desire to have intimate contact.

- When achieving orgasm becomes a habit both lovers tend to concentrate more on their own feelings and sensations and on the desire to make a good impression on each other (i.e. arouse the other) than on sincere feelings of love. This can lead to inauthentic behaviour and a break-down of trust.

- A woman can feel insecure if her man does not ejaculate. She might think that it is her fault, that she is not able to bring her man to orgasm.

- A man can feel a sense of duty to ejaculate. If he doesn't ejaculate he might feel insecure and isolate himself wrapped up in his own fears. As a result his body might become unable to function in a healthy sexual manner.

- When orgasm doesn't happen partners tend to feel less loved.

Now, look deep into yourself. Why do you believe in this idea?

Maybe because of these reasons:

- You feel like you always want an orgasm.
- You feel good at the moment of orgasm.
- You believe that to orgasm is good for your health.
- You don't know anything about how having an orgasm actually affects your health and relationship in the future.
- You are afraid of feeling tension and discomfort in your body or feeling emotional frustration if you do not reach orgasm,
- You are afraid of losing your partner if you do not provide an orgasm.
- You do not believe that your partner is happy without orgasm even if he or she says otherwise.
- You do not ask for your partner's opinion on the subject.
- You follow what the majority of people say about orgasm.
- You believe the media and traditional doctors who advise us to always strive to reach orgasm.
- You do not research the subject but follow the instinctual impulses in the body to reach orgasm.
- You do not observe your own sensations and feelings and do not ask about your partner's sensations and feelings linked to orgasm.
- You feel that an orgasm is the greatest pleasure in life because you don't know any other sexual pleasures.
- You don't want to change your habit of reaching orgasm because to change takes effort.
- You do not want to complicate things and instead follow the easiest path which is having an orgasm.

The peak orgasm is only a function. The reflex of male ejaculation - and female ejaculation which women have developed these days - is just a result of stimulating certain nerve endings. Our body is full of 'buttons' to press to make us feel good. The problem arises later when we have become addicted to the use of such buttons in our brain and we end up like 'Pavlov's dogs'.

The female body biologically is not created for the purpose of ejaculation. On the contrary, its purpose is rather to save energy for the sake of having a baby. The female body is able to produce something similar to male ejaculation but only at certain times to help the sperm meet a ripe egg. When a woman has an expectation of achieving high arousal and orgasm she may experience emotional and physical irritation if she fails to achieve it. Peak orgasm in men is usually the end of their ability to continue lovemaking. Human beings have much more to offer in their sex lives than having peak orgasms.

The Unimacy approach maintains the following:

Your physiological orgasm does not contribute to you caring about your partner. The physiological orgasm can be avoided and your energy saved unless perhaps having a baby is the plan.

If you can let this understanding completely replace in your mind the old beliefs you will benefit straight away and instantly experience the following gains:

- You will no longer experience pressure or expectations on yourself and your partner during lovemaking.
- You will avoid energy loss and increase your vitality.
- You will pay more loving attention to your partner and receive more attention yourself.

- You will explore and develop more tools to use in physical love including a different type of orgasm which is longer lasting.
- You will enjoy your body's sensuality and a soul connection with your partner.
- You will feel a deeper sense of bonding, connection and respect in relation to your partner.

We need to have a clear understanding of the actions people perform when trying to achieve the sensation called in most sources of information 'orgasm'. We never clearly understand what we do when we try to protect our 'orgasm rights'. There are two consenting adults present when we engage in sex. However, the respect for the other person is often lost at the moment one partner drives him or herself towards the experiencing of the orgasmic sensation. Women suffer in this type of situation more often than men because of the more fragile nature of their bodies and their more sensitive psychology. The differentiation between the physiological orgasm and the 'valley orgasm' which I described earlier fundamentally changes our attitude towards sex.

Lovemaking Should End With An Intense, Overwhelming And Mind-Blowing Sensation

Even if you agree with the idea of avoiding physiological orgasm you can still believe that there should be some sort of 'completion' as a result of lovemaking. Obviously, if you desire this type of mind-blowing 'completion' you cannot for the moment think of anything but the physiological orgasm.

Firstly, let us analyse how this idea of the requirement for intense completion via orgasm got into your mind.

Maybe because:

- When you had this mind-blowing sensation for the first time you liked it.
- You created the sensation again, with a partner or alone (masturbating), and again you liked it.
- You got into the habit of having this sensation,
- You don't know what else could give you the same sense of pleasure.

Do you notice that the words "your partner" are absent from all the reasons for holding onto your need for the orgasmic sensation listed above? Your partner is not there. You are alone with your desire. You use your partner's body to get what you desire, to achieve the physiological orgasm. Your actions again simply serve your body's instinctual drive. If your partner wants the same you are both serving your instinctual desires using each other's bodies.

Think about your hormones.

Scientific research has shown that any intense, overwhelming and mind-blowing sensation makes the human body produce the 'Drug Hormone' dopamine. Dopamine is released as a result of the anticipation of and then achievement of a goal, such as an orgasm. Because of the high rise in dopamine levels an orgasm produces it gives you a sense of pleasure the same way the intake of alcohol does.

The consequences of a sharp increase in dopamine production immediately followed by a sharp decline of the hormone is however not harmless. Such extreme changes in the body can cause fluctuations in the psyche and in our general life energy levels. After having an orgasm you want another orgasm and then another one... Even if you cannot... Just like as drug addict.

You will benefit from considering the following:

Physical love has no emotional or energetic end. Just the opposite; it creates a continuous balance emotionally and energetically!

If you hold this belief you will become a relaxed and happy person. You will be as energised by lovemaking as if you had been drinking fresh, pure water from the mountains. You will physically disconnect from your partner only because you feel you have fully expressed yourself and are loved and sexually balanced as your physical, sexual hunger is satiated.

One Should Be Highly Aroused During Sex

Intense arousal is like a marathon for the body. During a long period of high arousal the human body produces an enormous amount of dopamine. The heart rate is greatly increased and because of this there are cases of heart attack due to this high arousal and to orgasm.

Why do you hold the belief that there is a need for high arousal? I will tell you what my clients have told me. Probably, like them, you think that:

- Without high arousal you and your partner cannot have orgasms.
- You feel good when you are highly aroused.
- You feel more connected to your partner when you experience high arousal.
- You feel that your partner is more strongly connected to you if he or she experiences high arousal.

It is wonderful that you think about your partner, that you want to feel connected and secure in this connection. However, the physical body always strives for balance and comfort. It wants affection, but with less stress than it experiences when a lot of dopamine is produced.

And there are other hormones you can produce. The physical body loves them. They create calmness, lightness, complete happiness and peace. These hormones are the 'Bonding Hormone' oxytocin and the endorphins, the hormones of child-like joy. These hormones provide a deeper sense of security. But to experience these equally satisfying hormones you need to change your beliefs about the importance of orgasm in the sense this word is generally understood.

You need to become aware of another natural part of you:

We can help each other maintain the sexual energy flow at a more gentle and comfortable level of intensity during the whole time of lovemaking by creating sweet waves throughout our entire bodies.

Instead of intense arousal you create in your body sweet waves of gentler arousal. By doing this you invite your partner to do the same. You both maintain clarity in the mind. You both maintain a peaceful joyful mood. You constantly observe and enjoy the sexual energy rise and fall. You develop the ability to notice how your life energy changes after lovemaking, how it increases or decreases. Accordingly you can fine-tune your energy flow during your next lovemaking session.

Look at this from a purely practical perspective like you would in business. You have to know where your business is going: have you had more profit than losses? You improve what you do to increase your 'profit'.

Sexual energy is that endless stream from which we can always scoop up more strength, health and balance when we understand how to get in the flow.

One Should Be Highly Aroused
Before Engaging In Sex

A lot of men and women feel offended and even accuse their partners of a lack of love for them if their partner is struggling with physical arousal before intercourse. Women often judge their male partners the way a farmer judges his bull when he wants him to mate and puts the beast in front of the cows!

Men do the same: if women do not get wet, men feel that they are not loved, not desired or wanted as lovers.

High arousal before engaging in sex creates the risk of premature ejaculation in men. This is what every bull does – ejaculates quickly. High arousal also creates a quick orgasm in women. During my many years of sex coaching I have had a lot of male clients complaining about their wives reaching orgasm very quickly. After that the women did not want to continue lovemaking but simply helped their men to ejaculate. These men missed loving affection. Men do need affection too, surprising as this may seem to some people!

To require arousal before penetration creates in all of us a damaging cocktail of expectation, fear, complexes and tension.

This myth of the need for arousal before making love comes from the following assumptions:

- If the penis is not fully erect it is not possible to have intercourse or sex.

- If the vagina is not aroused properly it is more difficult to insert the penis.

These assumptions are not true. You can have sex, including intercourse, when the penis is not aroused fully, even not aroused at all and also when a woman's vagina is not wet or fully open.

There is an expression: "Appetite comes with eating". The same applies to arousal. I do not mean physiological arousal which is raised by stimulating certain body reflexes. Very often in long term relationships mechanical physiological stimulation does no longer work while emotional connection and romantic touch might work. If we start to touch each other with love our bodies will start to experience warm feelings and then waves of arousal. However this takes time and it has to be genuine feelings of love, it cannot be forced or faked.

Your new belief will sound like this:

Both partners can have sex, including intercourse, being mildly aroused or not aroused at all.

Sometimes if you are too aroused before starting intercourse it is better to bring your arousal down to a soft comfortable level to make it possible to connect emotionally with your partner. Your genitals can touch as if they were hugging. The genitals should be treated with delicacy and extreme patience.

This more balanced approach gives both partners a chance to synchronise their feelings and movements and create simultaneous waves of arousal, which in turn generates more desire. In this case nothing is forced, everything is happening without any pressure or discomfort. Both partners are meeting each other where they are as if walking hand in hand. Their mood and energy is similar, they feel a sense of oneness.

Sex Should Be Spontaneous, Overwhelming And Passionate (Hot)

This belief destroys a lot of relationships. Scientists claim that passionate love cannot last forever for reasons of a biochemical nature. The human body is programmed to adapt to and become used to stimulants. Sociological studies have shown that most divorces occur after 2-4 years of marriage. People are not aware that passionate sex risks to exhaust them and their relationship.

Unfortunately most people view the absence of passion as an absence of love. They can be chasing the feeling of passion all their lives and it is like chasing a phantom. It comes and it goes. While waiting for these spontaneous bursts - that will eventually appear less and less frequently - a lot of wonderful couples that are really made for each other suddenly find themselves losing the physical attraction. This leads to a tragedy in the relationship.

This idea of sexual passion strongly occupies people's minds because:

- Most men and women believe that a passionate behaviour is a sign of the chemistry of love.
- They believe this is how the body behaves naturally.
- They think men and women are programmed to behave in a passionate way.
- They think men and women like to behave passionately because it's thrilling.

- They believe sexual passion will make them feel more desired by their partners.
- They think passionate sex gives confidence and makes us sexually attractive.
- The media, doctors and psychologists maintain and promote the idea of passionate sex.
- There are no resources available to teach men and women a different sexual behaviour.

You do not need to exhaust yourself by looking for passion or fear the lack of it if your passion is gone. Instead you can have true love.

Your new belief to work on is:

The process of making love is an act that requires learning, planning and creativity.

Will you stay employed or have a successful business if you go to your office spontaneously? Or if you passionately touch your computer and then, being overwhelmed, type something extravagant to your boss? It can be fun maybe... But what your boss wants from you is a different type of attitude for things to work well.

Our physical body and its senses are connected to the brain, which is our boss. We can easily get upset if we or someone else is not caring towards our body and does not know what makes it happy. Why do you think a lot of couples stop making love after a few years of marriage? Why, as a result of that, do they argue more? Why do 50% of all married couples get divorced? Why is there such a high turn-over of lovers in the gay community? Still, most of them when they got together had passionate sex and even loved each other.

Physical love is a very delicate activity. To become good at making love last takes time and effort. It also requires a period of study and practice similar to the study of dancing or playing a musical instrument. The more effort, thoughts and feelings you put into it, the more you master your bodily movements, the more you enjoy dancing or playing music the better you will be at it. It is the same when it comes to physical love.

Five Main Unimacy Beliefs

I would like to repeat again five of the main Unimacy beliefs. Then I would like to continue bringing to your mind ideas that will help you create a happy love life for the rest of your life.

Look at these beliefs again and let them settle deep in your mind!

Your physiological orgasm does not contribute to you caring about your partner. The physiological orgasm can be avoided and your energy saved unless perhaps having a baby is the plan.

Physical love has no emotional or energetic end. Just the opposite; it creates a continuous balance emotionally and energetically!

We can help each other maintain the sexual energy flow at a more gentle and comfortable level of intensity during the whole time of lovemaking by creating sweet waves throughout our entire bodies.

Both partners can have sex, including intercourse, being mildly aroused or not aroused at all.

The process of making love is an act that requires learning, planning and creativity.

You can widen your horizons related to physical love by taking part in the Unimacy programs to learn practical techniques. And you need to be careful when confronted with many of the mainstream ideas. They can be very distracting and detrimental to lasting sexual happiness.

Other Mainstream Ideas About Sex

There are twelve other mainstream ideas that I can think of that can be interpreted differently by the partner's. Some of them are relevant only to heterosexual people. In most cases partners do not discuss these ideas with each other which means they can live in a state of misunderstanding for years. Obviously it makes their sexual relationship difficult. These conventional ideas include:

- A man should always bring a woman to orgasm first before having his own orgasm.
- A man should have a big penis to be able to satisfy a partner sexually.
- Before penetration a man should always spend time on foreplay.
- Foreplay is good for the woman because it makes her more aroused.
- A woman should seduce her partner and make him desire her madly sexually.
- A good lover is someone who has had a lot of lovers.
- Sexual games, sex toys and erotic films help sustain the relationship.
- Sex is all about genitals and erogenous zones.
- Sex means intercourse.

- The man should be active and the woman should be relaxed and be taken by her man.
- Sexual positions provide a variety of sensations during sex and make sex better.
- The best time for sex is night time.

A Man Should Always Bring A Woman To Orgasm First Before Having His Own Orgasm

Why is this belief so popular among men? The reasons are:

- It makes the man feel confident in being a good lover.
- It gives the man a feeling of being a good person when he does not try to get his own orgasm first.
- It makes him believe that the woman will love him for what he is doing for her.

In my practice I have met a lot of men that could not understand why their wives didn't like it when they tried to bring them to orgasm first.

Most women have a very sensitive vagina. When a woman has reached orgasm her vagina can quickly cool down ('dry'). If her man wants to have an orgasm for himself he often needs to perform a rigid, energetic entry into her vagina. A woman after orgasm experiences a state of euphoria, love and happiness that can be reduced if her man continues to rub her vagina for a long time. If he is not able to ejaculate soon after bringing her to orgasm she will try to help him by the same rigid movements. Many women experience unpleasant and even painful sensations in their vaginas when doing this. Sometimes it can even lead to severe irritation in a woman's genitals.

Vaginismus is considered to be a sexual problem in women that needs medical attention. Women develop this vaginal spasm because of men's actions, in particular connected to orgasm. Women can heal the vaginismus only if their men are willing to treat their vaginas lovingly and with care.

So if a man brings his woman to orgasm first he needs to be aware of how long he can continue intercourse without hurting her. He needs to stop intercourse and balance his energy in other ways if his woman experiences physical or emotional discomfort.

I would like men to pay attention to the fact that often when a woman has reached orgasm she starts to push her man to orgasm. A man can develop premature ejaculation because of this. The other fact is that a lot of women pretend to have reached orgasm. They know that if they are aroused it will help their men to achieve orgasm more quickly and save their genitals from irritation. Many women even pretend to have achieved orgasm very quickly so they can start to push their men towards orgasm even faster.

Here is the new idea for you to bear in mind and practise:

Both partners are synchronised in movements, breathing, touches and level of arousal. They are attentive to each other's needs and fulfil these by giving each other signs of what they want.

A Man Should Have A Big Penis To Be Able To Satisfy A Partner Sexually

A lot of sources of information recognise how stupid this idea is. However in my practice I still meet a lot of men that are very concerned about the size of their penises. They are scared of approaching women because they believe they have small penises. They avoid all relationships because of this belief. Some of them think about having an operation or have already had one to enlarge their penis. The media can do a lot of harm to people!

I understand that even if you are a man who has decided to become a conscious lover and you are happy not to think about your genitals but about the person you are with, you could still have a thought in the back of your mind that you cannot give to your partner the best experience if the size of your penis is not sufficient to penetrate the vagina deeply.

Firstly, I have to remind you that a lot of women suffer from pain in their vaginas during intercourse because even an average sized penis can be too big for them. Secondly, the media presents men as sexually attractive if they have big penises. In reality women rarely care about what the male genitals look like. Every woman I have taught or spoken with about her sexual experiences appreciated more the skill of her partner to penetrate her body gently, slowly and carefully. If a woman is highly aroused and the vagina becomes very open and wet there are techniques and sexual positions to help her partner create a sense of deep and tight penetration.

Obviously there are women who have developed a desire for powerful stimulation of their genitals and who like when the penis is big and hard. These types of women can make men very exhausted when having sex with them. Men don't need to avoid this type of women. They can be wonderful people but have somehow reduced their sensitivity through the habit of this rough practice. It could be that these women would love to change but simply haven't had a chance. A man can help such a woman by helping her relax more, retrain herself and become more sensual, gentle and loving. A man can help this kind of woman find deeper happiness and greater fulfillment in sex. All people are naturally loving and gentle. Men and women today are working hard and often get tired. In some ways the rough way of practising sexuality is like a drug or a form of stress relief. Care, acceptance and love towards these types of women will open up a new sexual world to both partners.

So the new principle is:

Any bodyshape or form and any health condition in your partner is accepted and loved. Every body is a treasure for his or her partner.

Before Penetration A Man Should Always Spend Time On Foreplay

There is nothing wrong with having foreplay before intercourse. However, foreplay usually means to stimulate a woman in order to arouse her as a preparation for intercourse. Women expect foreplay from men for the following reasons:

- Foreplay can be a great pleasure for a woman.
- It makes her properly aroused before penetration and intercourse.

Obviously a man experiences himself to be a better lover if he can provide good foreplay. But men are constantly puzzled and anxious about how to perform 'foreplay'. This uncertainty regarding foreplay makes him clumsy and nervous and in this condition he definitely can't create physical comfort for his woman. It all ends up being potentially disastrous for the lovemaking and for creating a lasting relationship. The truth is that whatever he does today won't necessarily work tomorrow because the female body is changing in its sensations. This can lead to even more stress for the man and to more disappointment for his woman.

Because foreplay is viewed by most men as a purely physical stimulation to create in the female body a high level of arousal for the purposes of easy penetration, the woman often takes on a passive role. A lot of men perform foreplay as if they need to push certain buttons on the female body. They do the work, but the pleasure is still far away.

Sometimes women enjoy foreplay, sometimes not. Sometimes women get overexcited and reach orgasm during foreplay. In any case most women concentrate on their own sensations and if they reach orgasm they then push their man towards orgasm too. For many couples this type of practice becomes a habit and problems develop with premature ejaculation in the man.

But there is another form of foreplay where both partners are involved in lovemaking together and mutually. They can simultaneously touch each other in many different ways as well as have intercourse. Intercourse can be started and stopped at any time and several times during the lovemaking. The partners can even engage in penetration at the very beginning using lubricant or massage oil to prepare the genitals for a smooth and comfortable connection. They can then interrupt penetration and continue with foreplay. This way a man always receives feedback from his woman so that he knows what she desires at a particular moment of the lovemaking.

The new principle to keep in mind is:

Both partners before, during and after penetration create continuous and mutual lovemaking actions where foreplay is a love play between both of them all the time. Female arousal can be awakened during penetration through special techniques based on care, trust and relaxation. The partners create a 'dance of love' together, a sequence of romantic touches (penetration is a form of touch too) to maintain the flow of happy energy.

Foreplay Is Good For The Woman
Because It Makes Her More Aroused

There is nothing wrong with the above statement if foreplay is part of lovemaking and not just a stimulation of the female body. Unfortunately in many cases foreplay eventually becomes a repetitive sequence of actions performed by the man that doesn't arouse but instead irritates his woman. There are no mutual 'sparks', no communication, no development and no expansion.

Men tend to be less creative than women. Sexuality is feminine in its nature as it is an art. I have found in my practice and through my own experiences that it is better if during foreplay the woman is the leader. When a woman starts touching first and involves her man in the 'dance of love' she creates a special atmosphere and a gentle and gradual arousal. It is a beautiful and exciting process for both.

Any woman can experience real joy and the opportunity to create the right arousal in her body when she acts herself. It gives her the pleasure of expressing her own sexual nature and cultivating her inner sense of beauty and artistry. This way she can prepare her body much better for intercourse. She can help her man to reduce his sexual frustration and impatience to enter her body before she is ready for it.

This is your new belief:

The woman is a better leader in foreplay than the man because of the feminine nature of creativity and art. This means the woman should lead.

Obviously Damaging Ideas

The next three ideas I find clearly damaging for any relationship. These beliefs can be forgotten if you decide never to allow yourself to think this way again.

The damaging ideas are:

- **A woman should seduce her partner and make him desire her madly sexually.**
- **A good lover is someone who has had a lot of lovers.**
- **Sexual games, sex toys and erotic films help to sustain the relationship.**

All three ideas have nothing to do with love.

Seduction was a survival tool for women for generations; it may be classed as manipulation. Manipulation is said to be the last resort for the powerless which means many women who feel they have no power still use it at present. Female seductive behaviour is then reinforced by the media as the way a woman can get a partner and keep him.

Any independent woman who wants to truly love and be loved knows that she cannot always behave seductively. What's more, she feels like a sex object if her partner wants her to behave like that.

A lot of wives shut down sexually when they turn from young playful girls into mothers and serious professionals while their husbands want them to dress up seductively in sexy outfits, watch porn or perform sexual acts like those enacted in erotic films. Sexual games and erotic films often present a woman as the man's sex toy. How could this help sustain a relationship?

It's the same with having a lot of lovers.

What kind of lasting experiences can one gain from that? Every new lover usually provides the same circle of sexual experience: falling in love, having a lot of passionate sex with a physiological orgasm, getting bored, tired, disappointed and then looking again for a new lover. Having a lot of lovers can be a waste of valuable time and energy. It is hardly likely to give you an experience of love. Love develops with time and when two partners work together on their relationship.

Men and women who are counting lovers, (i.e. who are 'pick-uppers') can often be very selfish individuals. They are also more likely to develop a 'consumer' attitude towards other people's bodies and energies. They are less able to love and connect, which takes time, and so are unable to sustain a relationship. Many people in this group see sex as a physical performance for their ego.

The important thing is not how many lovers you have had but what experiences you gathered from these relationships. What you have understood and learned from these lovers. How you have changed and how you have developed as a lover.

Sexual stimulants also contribute to creating a consumer attitude towards the physical body, your own and others. They take men or women away from fulfilling and lasting lovemaking, reduce the body's sensitivity and eliminate the need to understand the sexual partner and their subtleties. They create a world of dreams, similar to drug use and can even lead to sexual violence, intentional or not.

Unfortunately the media does not present experiences of love and connection through the physical body and through sexual arousal. Just the opposite; it presents the mechanisms of abuse.

Instead of the above ideas it is more conducive to a deeply satisfying love life to adopt the following attitudes:

A woman can freely express sexual love. She is open to love sexually and able to connect with her partner physically and emotionally. She enjoys it when her partner appreciates her either through touch or through watching her.

We are all lovers for life. We need to be the only one for each other, the first and the last one.

All actions during lovemaking are natural. They are the romantic discovery of each other's bodies again and again, melting into each other's sexual heat.

Five Ideas Disadvantageous To A Happy Relationship

- **Sex is all about genitals and erogenous zones.**
- **Sex means intercourse.**
- **The man should be active and the woman should be relaxed and be taken by her man.**
- **Sexual positions provide variety of sensations during sex and make sex better.**
- **The best time for sex is night time.**

Sex is all about genitals and erogenous zones.

When our genitals are touched we feel instantly a strong and pleasant energy in this part of our body. Men and women think that if they are focused on genitals and erogenous zones they will reach physiological orgasm easier. This is true if you are looking only to satisfy your sexual instinct.

If you are a 'new man' or a 'new woman' who wants to create a stable and happy sexual relationship you want to create something special in your sex life. Touching each other's genitals and erogenous zones is of course important to maintain sexual arousal. The body tends to get used to sensations however. Desensitisation is our survival tool: we stop feeling hot, cold, pain... Touching body parts as sensitive as genitals is a very delicate matter. When we repeatedly touch them in the same way the sensitivity fades. You may not think that when your genitals are touched you lose sensitivity there, but you do. After a time you need stronger stimulation in order to maintain arousal.

By focusing too much on genitals and erogenous zones men and women do not develop the sensuality of the whole body. Gradually their sensual potential is reduced. This often leads to increased stimulation of genitals and it becomes a vicious circle: the harder and faster the genitals are stimulated the more dramatically their sensitivity decreases. And not only in the current sexual act. It has an impact on future acts too because we have a physical memory. Focusing on genitals creates a sense of routine, boredom and physicality.

Of course we need to pay a lot of attention to genitals and erogenous zones during lovemaking. Touching and being touched in these areas of our bodies makes us feel sexually wanted. It has a tremendous impact on our confidence, on our sense of worthiness and well-being.

However, it is beneficial to understand that:

The whole body can love and be loved as a sexual body. The whole body can be an erogenous zone. Every part of the human body can give us an immense wealth of sensations. Physical love is a love towards the body as a whole.

A lot of men may think that their shoulders for example are not as sensual as their penises in terms of increasing their sexual arousal. Women on the other hand are more likely to think that any part of their bodies is able to respond to a special kind of touch and able to bring even more arousal. Sometimes other parts of the female body respond even better than the erogenous zones and genitals.

Why is this so? The answer is simply that women more often than men connect touch with the emotion of love and this in itself is deeply arousing. If a man develops his emotional side in connection with touch he too can expand his body's erogenous zones to include the whole body.

In my many years of sexual teaching and coaching practice with men I have had this proven to me over and over. Every man who had a coaching session with me could never forget this wonderful experience of his body's wholeness. Women need to learn how to help their men become more sensual.

Unfortunately these days many women are doing the opposite, i.e. they develop a more masculine behaviour in sex. In my programs I give step-by-step guidance on how to develop higher sensuality. By the word "sensuality" I mean the inseparable union of the physical body with its five senses and the emotional mind with its loving images, feelings and thoughts.

Sex means intercourse.

Imagine that intercourse is not possible (due perhaps to illness, pregnancy, etc...). What would you do? How long would you be patiently happy to live your life without intercourse? Wouldn't you look 'over the fence, where the grass is greener' looking for another potential sex partner? Wouldn't you feel unloved?

The belief that sex means intercourse makes your partner obliged to have intercourse when he or she just wants a physical sign of affection. It's very common that couples cease any romantic or sensual contact if intercourse is not regularly on the agenda.

This belief creates a great fear of rejection and of losing the partner when intercourse ceases. One partner is frightened to initiate physical contact, the other fears to be left for another sexual partner who provides intercourse readily. Nobody will provide intercourse 'on request' however. It is not that simple. People often mistakenly take the first passionate stage of a new relationship for a promise of 'hot sex on demand'. When people get older they find it less of a problem to make love without intercourse.

Though it is very important to develop new, healthier attitudes towards physical love when your are young as it will influence your entire life for the better. It will help you avoid many of the pitfalls that the old myths create when it comes to the sexual habits of couples.

The new, healthier attitude is:

Intercourse is not the one and only important element of physical love. Other forms of body-to-body contact can give just as much happiness and energy and create as much of a sense of love and closeness as intercourse does.

Other forms of touching genitals without having intercourse raise soft and pleasant energies and create romantic and loving feelings. They help to overcome the desire to orgasm, especially in men. They can replace intercourse. Other ways of genital contact can create deep trust in the female body and help the woman feel more love through the touch of her lover. We can create a feeling of deep appreciation by learning new ways of touching each other without the need for intercourse. In general the results we experience all depend on how our genitals are touched.

I do believe though that everyone is able to have intercourse with his or her partner every day. It all depends on how we have intercourse. For example, among my clients there was a couple who made love with intercourse on the day the wife went to the hospital to have a baby. There was a couple where the husband was disabled, paralysed from the waist down with no sensation in his penis. Even so the couple had intercourse and the husband even experienced orgasm, which I call a mental orgasm.

Women tend to leave out intercourse more than men. In my programs for women I give step-by-step guidance on how to enjoy intercourse every time your man wants it... And he wants it all the time...

The man should be active and the woman should be relaxed and be taken by her man.

This traditional belief is still widespread among men and women. Unfortunately it creates an opportunity for the woman to blame the man for her sexual unhappiness and put unrealistic expectations on him. The man develops fear and tiredness; making love becomes hard work for him.

Many teachings and sex advice have claimed that a passive, relaxed woman gets more easily aroused. A lot of modern advice on how to attract women claim that an active man is viewed by the woman as more desirable because this way she will feel his masculine power. Sadly, men and women are both hooked on the many games they play in sex. They have no awareness that in the long run their relationship is bound to collapse as a result of the illusions they have built related to the opposite sex.

A lot of wonderful men who are gentle and caring are afraid to start relationships because they do not feel confident being these 'active men'. They are especially nervous when thinking about how to bring women to orgasm.

What about women? This dangerous belief has a lot of wonderful, gentle and caring women waiting for the men they feel attracted to, to begin initiating physical contact. They fear that if they initiate contact themselves they will be viewed by the men as flighty, unreliable and not truly loving potential partners. So whilst good women are waiting, good men are procrastinating.

Today men and women are gaining more equality. A lot of women do initiate sex. However, this female initiative is often simply a sign to men that they want to have sex and still not a conscious initiative to nurture men, to help them relax and relieve them of their 'responsibility' to satisfy women.

Men have changed. A lot of men are intellectual and intelligent, cultured and well-mannered. They are not happy with just biologically programmed instinctual sexual activity. They are no longer happy with playing the dominating role and conquering women. A lot of modern men have developed a deeper understanding of sexuality and want to find a deeper meaning in sex. They need women to help them develop a more nurturing attitude towards their bodies as they feel ashamed of their sex drive. They cannot dominate the female body and act on instinctive impulses without thinking as they once did.

I have worked with a lot of young men who are still virgins at the age of 30 because they feel vulnerable with women in an intimate situation. They worry about a lot of things when they are with women: their own behaviour, their attitude towards women and the consequences of the sexual act. Women need to change their passive attitude and help men get in touch with their nurturing and caring side instead of demanding transitory passion and sexual satisfaction.

It is more helpful to develop this more balanced attitude:

Both partners can initiate sex. Both partners should touch and nurture each other's bodies mutually.

Sexual positions provide a variety of sensations during sex and make sex better.

In opposition to all sexuality teachings, including spiritual practices like Tantra and Taoist teachings that all present and advocate different sexual positions, my own experience and that of a lot of other people - especially women - has shown me that merely changing sexual positions is not always a good thing. It can break the established emotional and physical connection between partners and reduce or completely interrupt the sexual arousal. It can even create a strong sense of disappointment and resentment.

The idea of changing sexual positions usually comes from the desire to keep a fading level of arousal alive. It is not aimed at creating a stronger emotional bond but merely wants to physically stimulate the arousal. Partners looking for new sexual positions can lose a sense of intimacy and love. This is my deep belief and it has been proven to me many times. After some time a changing of positions does no longer work - as nothing works for long if it is only a search for novelty. Changing positions can also be physically exhausting.

The idea was born out of a lack of imagination and a lack of emotional involvement during lovemaking. This happens when men and women rely solely on physical activity in their search for satisfaction and fulfilment.

Why do doctors and sex therapists widely recommend changing sexual positions?

What do most doctors know? Do any of them have imagination needed to know how to love physically, how to touch, how to nourish the body? As far as I know from my research most professionals follow mainstream beliefs about sexual arousal and satisfaction.

What about the media? Here the hunt for a good story means it is mostly not possible to show an emotional connection. Sexual positions on the other hand are good for 'the show'.

The new belief is this:

Bodies do not need novelty. Bodies are involved in synchronised movements. The partners do as much as they want and are able to do physically in order to feel emotional closeness.

The bodies relax and merge with each other in comfortable positions. The partners might use only one position. The bodies reach an experience similar to that of travelling in the same boat through the ocean. The ocean of love is the main focus.

The best time for sex is night time.

When night comes most people feel tired and their energies are low. They will mostly have quick sex before sleep. This results in poor erection in men and leads to premature ejaculation. If the woman is tired she will push the man towards ejaculation. Sex can become a rare, boring and short routine, a purely physical activity before falling asleep.

People tend to associate sex with the night time because:

- Things seem more romantic at night.
- At night we somehow seem more beautiful and sexually attractive.
- The media presents sex at night time as more romantic.
- This is often the only time people have the opportunity to have sex.

If couples would plan their life properly and if they would believe that their sexual relationship is a very important part of their lives they will agree with me that the best time for lovemaking is the day time.

It is better to think:

The best time for lovemaking is day time.

Realistically love making is possible straight after work, before going to work and on weekends any time of the day. Then couples can also make love before going to bed. However at night lovemaking should be different and both partners physical and energetic abilities should always be taken into consideration.

Seventeen Beliefs And Unimacy Principles

1. Your physiological orgasm does not contribute to you caring about your partner. The physiological orgasm can be avoided and your energy saved unless perhaps having a baby is the plan.
2. Physical love has no emotional or energetic end. Just the opposite; it creates a continuous balance emotionally and energetically!
3. We can help each other maintain the sexual energy flow at a more gentle and comfortable level of intensity during the whole time of lovemaking by creating sweet waves throughout our entire bodies.
4. Both partners can have sex, including intercourse, being mildly aroused or not aroused at all.
5. The process of making love is an act that requires learning, planning and creativity.
6. Both partners are synchronised in movements, breathing, touches and level of arousal. They are attentive to each other's needs and fulfil these by giving each other signs of what they want.
7. Any body-shape or form and any health condition in your partner is accepted and loved. Every body is a treasure for his or her partner.
8. Both partners before, during and after penetration create continuous and mutual lovemaking actions where foreplay is a love play between both of them all the time. Female arousal can be awakened during penetration through special techniques based on care, trust and relaxation. The partners create a 'dance of love' together, a sequence of romantic touches (penetration is a touch too) to maintain the flow of happy energy.

9. The woman is a better leader in foreplay than a man because of the feminine nature of creativity and art. This means the woman should lead.

10. A woman can freely express sexual love. She is open to loving sexually, and able to connect with her partner physically and emotionally. She enjoys it when her partner appreciates her either through touch or through watching her.

11. We are all lovers for life. We need to be the only one for each other, the first and the last one.

12. All actions during lovemaking are natural. They are the romantic discovery of each other's bodies again and again, melting into each other's sexual heat.

13. The whole body can love and be loved as a sexual body. The whole body can be an erogenous zone. Every part of the human body can give us an immense wealth of sensations. Physical love is a love towards the body as a whole.

14. Intercourse is not the one and only important element of physical love. Other forms of body-to-body contact can give just as much happiness and energy and create as much of a sense of love and closeness as intercourse does.

15. Both partners can initiate sex. Both partners should touch and nurture each other's bodies mutually.

16. Bodies do not need novelty. Bodies are involved in synchronised movements. The partners do as much as they want and are able to do physically in order to feel emotional closeness.

17. The best time for lovemaking is day time.

Planting these 17 Unimacy principles deeply into your mind will tremendously change your attitude towards sex. It will free you from worries about how to impress and perform and what to achieve as a lover. Though you still need to develop a lot of skills, practise them and expand your creative romantic imagination through learning new techniques and through listening to and watching your partner. You have to become a gift to your lover.

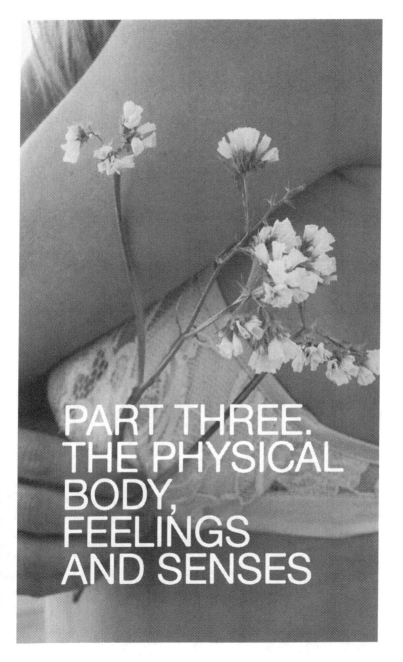

PART THREE.
THE PHYSICAL
BODY,
FEELINGS
AND SENSES

Self-Learning And Self-Balancing
Versus Masturbation

Many men and women are not able to communicate clearly to their partners what they feel in their bodies during intimacy. They cannot express themselves through touch. Often people don't understand their own bodies, neither are they able to understand the needs of their partner's body. This lack of physical understanding creates emotional tension in the relationship.

I believe that everyone has to develop their sexuality through solo practice first to gain full control of their sex drive and expand the loving and sensual capacity of their bodies. Sexuality has not been accepted culturally in many societies. As a result there is no education in place to teach us how to deal with our instincts, how we can self-regulate and balance our bodies when we experience sexual urges. Respect and love towards our own physical body, an exploration of its capacity to sense, feel and enjoy touch is alien to most people. Women by nature are more connected to and more in touch with their bodies. For men the body is often an unknown land in terms of sensuality.

Working with many single men and women I know that it is not easy for most people to touch themselves for the purposes of learning. Though many men and women masturbate. Some people don't feel uncomfortable with masturbation. Others after masturbating (as many of my clients have reported) experience a sense of shame and guilt as well as physical tiredness and even a sense of emotional emptiness. Masturbation is generally a desire to release biologically programmed sexual tension. Most men and women know of only one way to relieve this tension: through physiological orgasm. If they have a sexual partner to help them get this release through having sex, orally, by hand or through other stimulation, they probably won't masturbate as often. A lot of people masturbate in front of their partners however. It makes them feel stronger arousal and this in turn can arouse their partners. Yet masturbation and watching someone masturbate brings out our most basic instincts. Whether you use your own hand, your partner's body or a toy it is still masturbation, as generally your aim is to relieve physiological sexual tension in the body. A lot of men and women try to reach orgasm quickly while masturbating 'to finish it off'. All this leads to a desensitising of their bodies and reduces their ability to engage emotionally. It results in premature ejaculation in men and a quick orgasm in women. It can cause a kind of 'disability' in you as a lover.

The practice of self-learning and self-balancing on the other hand is a preparation for a fulfilling love life with your partner. It allows safe exploration of your senses, an expansion of your sensuality and it develops the emotional and physical connection with your own body.

I have created programs for sexual self-exploration that will guide you step-by-step through the body's sensations. The human body is like the terrain of a huge country. It has a beautiful sensual landscape, but it takes time to get to know this landscape well.

When you are caring about and knowledgeable of your own body's sensuality, you are caring about your partner's body too.

Touching yourself with the intention to explore, you will find out so many things that you never imagined about the sensuality of the different parts of your body. As you receive and give touch to yourself you start to understand more clearly what kind of touch can arouse, relax, nourish and make someone feel special.

You will also activate in your brain the connection between touch and the emotion created by that touch. You will begin to understand the main principles underlying the way your sensual and sexual body operates during the process of touch. This is important for you to be able to achieve intimacy with your partner.

You will find out what parts of your body are most sensitive and able to give you strong sensations if your partner touches you there in a particular way. You will know what type of touch is less pleasant to you, not arousing sexual energy even if that part of your body is generally considered an erogenous zone. Some touches can have a ticklish effect on you and can make you laugh. Some touches can be really unpleasant and cause you to feel irritation, anxiety, fear, pain, frustration or even tiredness. It is very important for you to explore all of this and to let your partner know what kind of touch you enjoy and where. Let your partner know which part of your body to touch and how to touch it in order to create within you different emotions of love, security, peace, joy, happiness, trust, care and other positive and loving feelings.

This exploration of your own body is important. Not only for the sake of experiencing your own pleasure. It is important because your sensations, emotions and feelings will affect all your actions towards the body of your lover. A happy person touches differently than someone who experiences irritation or pain. It is your responsibility to educate yourself and your partner. He or she cannot know how to touch you if you don't know it yourself. There is no way for you to become a good lover unless you discover your own body sensations.

Differences Between Men And Women

There are significant physiological and emotional differences between men and women due to their natural biological purpose. These differences need to be understood and addressed by both partners. It is vital for the stability of the relationship. Misunderstanding and ignoring these differences lead to alienation, avoidance of physical contact, resentment, irritation and even disease. Subtle and careful learning of all the aspects of the feminine and masculine nature results in a knowing of the correct way of acting towards each other and helps to create true sexual happiness.

While reading this chapter I advise you to refer to your common sense. Try to understand your own body, listen to it, be honest with yourself and clearly define what makes your body feel good. Your body is a unique creation of nature that will never be repeated again in the exact same way. The same holds true for your partner's body. When your body meets your partner's body both bodies need to feel good. I want to highlight the similarities in all men as well as in all women but each couple has its own characteristics. In this chapter I am sharing my own observations of men and women. Do not consider this to be a generalisation of the sexes but more an expression of compassion and a desire to bring them together. You have the right to disagree with my opinion.

Women.

Women are emotional creatures. Women live from the heart. Also, they feel their bodies strongly. The female body is soft, flexible and craves sensual relaxation and pampering. Women long for a special kind of touch, the one she experiences when she is firmly held by her man as though he does not want to let her go. This gives her a sense of being wanted. At the same time these touches should be gentle, the man being careful not to hurt her physically. This gives her a sense of being loved and cared for. Many women would agree with this description. The female body does not always respond with arousal if a man simply manipulates her erogenous zones. Arousal in women, especially in long term relationships, is often dependant upon her emotional state, which if to be good needs three main factors to be present:

- She needs to feel safe and secure in relation to her natural purpose; giving birth and raising children, if she wants to have children.
- She needs to like the way her male partner's body looks.
- She needs to be touched by her man in the right way.

A woman can get sexually aroused at any age. She can maintain sexual arousal or be happy in the sexual act without strong excitation. Her physical capacity to feel sexual energy has no limitations. Her body is a rich sensual instrument. Correct touching of many parts of her body can give her great pleasure and excite the sexual energy. Unfortunately many women never feel this energy in their bodies. Poor sexual education, a puritan upbringing and negative sexual experiences generated by unpleasant male touch close the door to the rich world of female sexuality. Most women never come to discover the art of eroticism and sensuality. They might manage to reach orgasm but this is not the same as being sexually expressive.

Most women are deeply rooted in the belief that a man should do everything in bed and that the main pleasure of sex is the pleasure of orgasm which a man has to provide. Perhaps this female passivity was intended by nature: the man proclaims himself to be 'the master' of his woman's body and the woman feels that she belongs to the man that has entered her body. This way she feels devoted to her man and subconsciously focuses on carrying out the task of procreation. Surprisingly enough even today in the 21st century most women are still subconsciously programmed by this natural instinct to procreate when expressing their sexuality, even when they do not want to have children. In Eastern teachings the female orgasm is viewed as a call for the sperm to be released into the female body. Therefore most women want to achieve orgasm and they want their men to ejaculate. However, every woman has the ability to create a special world of love, healing and joy for her man and for herself. This ability is based on her inherent female artistry. A woman's skin has a special sensitivity, the female body is beautiful at any age. A woman can easily cope with her sexual arousal which gives her the opportunity to turn her sexuality into an oasis of peace and tranquillity for her man. The woman can increase the vitality of both her own and her partner's body as she is the source of a warm and soft energy.

Woman is a 'dancer' by nature. This means that all the movements of her body can be beautiful and sublime.

She can turn any sexual act into an art appealing to the soul not only to the body, awakening divine feelings and emotions towards herself, her partner and the whole world. As a result her man will also become a better, kinder, more peaceful person able to bring more goodness to the world. There is a sense of chastity inherent in the female body. It is not the kind of chastity proclaimed by religions: that a woman should preserve her virginity for the man who will marry her and that once married she should have sex purely for the purpose of procreation. Chastity for a woman is her outer and inner beauty that for her man creates a garden of love. A man takes pleasure from looking at her beautiful body, from feeling the warmth and softness of her vagina, from surrendering to her femininity, her calm, her peacefulness and tenderness. His natural instinct is tamed by being lost in the embrace of her mysterious and mystical feminine beauty. This view of female sexuality is quite different from the mainstream representation of female 'sexiness' that we see today on many magazines covers, in movies and in other sources of information on the subject of relationship and love. A married woman and mother will refuse to embody for her husband the image of a seductive and cutesy nymphomaniac. Yet media actively puts fear and doubt into the minds of women as to whether modest and gentle wives can stay sexually attractive to their husbands. There are huge amounts of women discussing the topic of sexuality in the Internet forums. They are asking: "What can I do if I don't want to have sex with my husband although I love him in every way?" I would advice these women: "Make your body a home for your man, a place where you are happy to invite him in and make him feel delight and rapture from your loving attitude towards his body!" Similar words are written in all the ancient teachings about love. What prevents modern women from following this advice? Maybe having the mind-set of a concubine? Throughout history women have been men's concubines. In the modern world we would proclaim that a woman has total freedom, but in fact she does not. She does not by nature possess the same abilities, and hence the possibilities and the power, to provide a living for herself as a man. It is clear that if she wants to have children it will be difficult for her to survive. For this reason the age-old psychology of the concubine dictates the sexual behaviour of many modern women. This is why many women lose interest in sex after getting married and if they do have sex they experience it as a duty. If they no longer experience the instinctual excitation in their bodies that they once felt before the marriage they decide they are not sexual any more, and sex is something they just put up with.

When a female body doesn't call for having a baby the woman can feel a lack of sexual desire. Any woman can notice that on certain days of the month she feels a strong sexual desire whilst on other days she doesn't. It is obvious that when getting older this biological need will diminish. However any woman can develop her sensuality by exploring her body. "What makes my body feel good during the sexual act? What do I need to do for this to happen? How can I teach my man to help me discover what gives me pleasure?" If a woman frees herself from the mind-set of a concubine she will find herself to be an equal sexual partner for her man. When she gives her man love through her body she transforms him from an ordinary man into a successful and strong man. The feminine energy of love is boundless like the ocean. This energy feeds the man and increases his vitality. To embrace this role as a woman in the male-female union gives her incredible confidence and self-esteem. She experiences herself as the man's equal half in the Union, but with a different objective. She experiences herself as the master of her own body, the hostess of her own life and the creator of her happiness by being the initiator in her and her man's love life. Love does not consist of requirements and expectations. Love is created by actions, in the same conscious and voluntary way a mother communicates with her child. Love is accompanied by patience, passion and the art of constructive dialogue. Women have all these qualities.

About female orgasm.

I am personally convinced that the female body is not created for physiological orgasm. Every orgasm results in a loss of energy and the female body is designed to accumulate energy. A woman's body is able to achieve physiological orgasm and can even have multiple orgasms. But there is not much dedication to love and constructive dialogue in the desire to have an orgasm. The desire to achieve orgasm can often make a woman appear selfish. The male orgasm is a natural process in the man's body due to his biological purpose. In women orgasm does not occur as easily as in men. For a woman to achieve orgasm she first has to convince herself that she should have one and, secondly, she needs to develop in her body the physiological mechanisms to achieve one. However, if achieving orgasm becomes a habit for her and, moreover, the dominant requirement for engaging in the sexual act, then the sexual act will have nothing to do with love. I don't see this type of development of female sexuality as being helpful in creating loving relationships. Reaching orgasm is like getting drunk, it makes the mind passive and dependent on a state of euphoria obtained not through hard work but simply by taking the drug. In this case the woman has developed a mechanism to obtain her drug. Also it results in her valuing her partner only for his ability to stimulate her to orgasm. When a woman puts all her effort into the desire to reach orgasm she gathers and directs all her major streams of energy to the genitals, especially the energy of the heart, her emotional centre. Many women scream and cry when they build up their arousal to the moment of orgasm. This crying and screaming takes a huge amount of life energy from the woman's body and can result in her afterwards experiencing depression, nervousness and tiredness. The truth is that at the moment of orgasm she doesn't feel a sense of love for her partner. If she would analyse what she feels during an orgasm, if she could record the state of her mind and body, she would clearly recognise feelings very different from the experience of love. These feelings are: a fear of losing her partner, a desire to get something from her partner, a sense of bewilderment and doubt about her partner's love for her. Many women have confessed to me that when they regained their balance after screaming and crying during orgasm they experienced a strong sense of shame. It seemed to them as if they had been doing something unworthy and dirty, as if they had been begging or pleading for something.

The feeling of love is a very light and happy state. It creates smiles not tears. When your attention is directed towards your partner instead of towards yourself you experience a different kind of arousal. It is a powerful vibration of happy energy flowing through your whole being. This vibration is caused by the presence of your partner very close to you. Women have also confessed to me that after having an orgasm they felt a strong desire to reject their partners. They had the experience of having their will seized and suppressed by the men and feeling as though their men owned them. I think this is the correct explanation to the state of the female psyche after orgasm. Scientists have identified the hormones causing this condition that are produced in large quantities by the body at the moment of strong arousal and orgasm. I have talked about this earlier in the book. Women need to learn how to manage their sexual arousal during the sexual act so that the dynamics of sexual arousal does not disrupt their equilibrium, nor that of their partners.

With regard to the physical body and its sensations, again, everything is in the woman's hands. The vagina is the part of her body a man enters. The act of intercourse is the main element of physical love. Without the act of coitus the expression of the feelings of love is not completed, the way a song is not completed without the last chord. The truth is, all battles between men and women take place around the act of coitus. Men always want to enter the vagina and ejaculate. It is their natural purpose for having sex. Assuming that a man could turn his brain off for a while and then turn it on again, what kind of desire would appear first in his head? I believe that the desire to enter his penis into the vagina occurs first, even before the desire to eat. If we assume that this is so, why wouldn't his woman help him cope with this natural instinct? Compare it to a situation where you are looking after children. When children are involved in interesting play they often forget about food. As a result they become moody and even sick. The caring mother will always prevent this situation by patiently stopping her children's play and feed them. The male sexual instinct has a similar character. It is difficult for a man to control his desire to enter a woman. He wants to do it as soon as possible and then he wants to ejaculate, the way children want to play and have no thought of dinner. A woman can take charge of her partner's sexual balance. By nature she is gifted with the ability to reduce male sexual tension. She does not need to follow the advice of modern sex therapists that recommend her to 'give her body to the man'. Instead she can 'embrace' him with her vagina.

Reading the above many women might mistrust my words. This is understandable. When a man feels extreme excitement he often does not listen to the woman's body and tries to release his sexual tension through ejaculation. He rubs the vagina in a rough manner and causes pain in the female tissues. The woman suffers from this unintentional violence towards her body. Changing the dynamics of male sexual behaviour is not done overnight. However, if a woman develops her sexuality, if she brings to the sexual act more creativity and takes more initiative, she can direct the masculine energy into a calm relaxed flow. By expressing gentleness, tenderness and care she can gradually teach her man a different sexual behaviour. A man who every day is 'fed' with love will become a better lover and a devoted and caring sex partner. Unfortunately most men live in a state of sexual hunger. I'll tell you more about this in the chapter about men...

Let us now return to the question of intimacy within the marriage. In many official medical and psychological textbooks we find the statement that young women are not very sexy. They are more focused on finding a good husband and then on having children and bringing them up. The words 'sexy woman' are commonly interpreted to mean a woman who often has a spontaneous desire for sexual contact, who likes to experience intense arousal in her body and then easily achieves orgasm. The same sources indicate that when a woman gets older she becomes sexier. This because becoming mature makes her see sex as an expression of her affection and love for her husband who is providing for her and her children, rather than a desire driven by the purpose of procreation.

Subsequently the question arises: "What if the man does not provide for the woman?" You will often hear from men: "All women want from men is money! Why can't they just love men as men?" I have heard resentful words from many men regarding the fact that their wives have sex with them only if they increase their family's welfare or buy presents.

Perhaps to some extent this is the truth. Again, many women might not agree with this view, although in many cases I doubt the sincerity of these women. A lack of sexual desire for a man who has achieved little is a natural reaction in women. In men the sexual desire is of a different nature. It comes from the attraction to the female body. A woman can also be attracted to the male body and use it to quench the sexual hunger arising in her body at times from her reproductive function. But in general this is not how it is for most women.

This said, even a woman with a husband who is a successful high achiever might not feel any sexual desire for him. He might treat her as a thing he owns and as a means to his own excitement.

And there is a third possibility. The man might be successful. He might respect and love his woman. Though if he is physically awkward and untidy, if he neglects looking after his body and touches the woman in an unpleasant way, she will still avoid sexual contact with him. And of course when there are children involved all the woman's energy will be directed towards them. All her love, her mental and bodily energy is now given to the children. Her body gives enormous amounts of touch to the bodies of her children. This satisfies her need for gentle touch and tenderness and becomes an expression of her chastity. Touching children is the most beautiful experience for a woman. At the same time touching the body of her husband can become even more unpleasant for her if this touching is intended to create high arousal and orgasm. In the mind of the woman-mother this type of physical contact is associated with the aggressive energy of desire and repression. During the initial romantic stage of a relationship she enjoys this energy because it is in line with her purpose to strengthen the man's desire to be with her, to marry and have children with her. Once she has consolidated her position as a wife and mother the purpose for expressing her sexuality changes. She now wants to experience more emotional love, she wants to relax and feel peaceful and balanced in her energy for the sake of her children. If the man doesn't change his attitude towards sex in accordance with her, if he is not following the path of her chastity, if he has not learnt to control his natural instinct and developed a meditative approach to intercourse, he might lose his wife as his sexual partner. The door to her body may close forever. And even worse, if the husband insists on sexual contact aiming to release his sexual tension by using her body, he will make her dislike him as a person. This is often exactly what happens in a marriage. After giving birth to her children a woman is subconsciously no longer relying solely on her natural reproductive sexuality. She has a sense that there is another side to sexuality that is loving and creative but she does not know how to express it. Her husband might hurt her by saying things like: "You are just not sexy...", coming from his expectation of his wife to seduce him, play with his body and want sex purely for physical pleasure. His wife may agree with his statement. She too might start thinking that she is not sexy as she does not feel a desire for sex in her body and no longer has an interest in playing seductive games. This can result in the woman remaining convinced for many years that something is sexually wrong with her. She will focus her life on many things but the physical love towards her husband will be excluded from the list. It is not difficult for her to live like this. Except for her experience of feeling a constant sense of guilt towards her husband and her fear that he will begin to insist on sexual contact or find another woman. This situation is common in many marriages. Men do not realise that every woman is sexual in her ability to open her body to love.

Modern young women often start to have sexual contact with men very early in their lives. They are not doing this as an expression of their natural procreative purpose nor out of love but in order to win the respect of their mates. The sexual behaviour of today's youth is a battle for credibility and respect, especially in developed countries. Young women are becoming like men sexually. They frighten men by their sexual demands to experience a purely physical pleasure. Many modern young women are sexually selfish and forceful. Countless women in bikinis talk on the Internet about 'multiple orgasms and female ejaculation'. I see all this as pretentious and business oriented. Unfortunately young women are poisoned by this kind of sexual propaganda. They masturbate a lot, have sex with many men as well as with their women-friends even when not being homosexual by nature. They often have sex being drunk or under the influence of drugs. They use all sorts of sexual stimulation, including porn and sex toys. It is no secret that most women start to stimulate themselves from the age of twelve. Modern women these days are not in a hurry to develop a serious loving relationship. They are convinced that they need extensive sexual experience (the more sexual partners, the better), a good career as well as a high income before they engage in a serious relationship. They are not aware that this attitude towards sex can destroy their sensuality and sexuality and make them incapable of loving. My system can help women become true lovers. A female body is designed for sexual dance, warmth, beauty, peace and love.

Men.

Men are logical creatures. Men live from their mind. They do not know their bodies well. A male body is not as flexible as a woman's. It always craves sexual arousal and orgasm. The man's whole body does not need much touching, he only longs for his penis to be touched. He touches his penis a lot himself. If possible, he would like his penis to be touched all the time, no matter who was touching it. If he has a woman in his life he does not want her to leave him simply because he needs her to touch his penis, whether with her hands, mouth, anus or vagina. Deep down he does not care about if he is wanted by his woman nor if he is loved and cared for. He just wants his penis to be erect. Many men would not agree with the above description but they should not be offended by it. It is not a criticism. The description is there for women to understand men better and this is what is biologically programmed into the male body and brain.

Nature has created everything in a very clever way. It has created in the man a constant need to discharge his sperm into a woman's body 'for the growth of the population', even if there is enough people in the world at this point. The woman is created 'not to let the man enter her'. The man is created 'to enter and inseminate the woman'. This represents a conflict of two opposites. A conflict that does not exist in animals because animal sexuality has only a reproductive function. People are much more complicated. Our sexual instinct is deeply connected with the psyche. Scientific research has proven that a man needs to have sexual contact or else he will get into a depressive mood and even worse, he may come close to suicide. But let's not talk about the extremes. Let's talk about reality, about the most common situation where men have sexual partners that they have sex with from time to time.

A male body always responds with arousal if a woman manipulates his erogenous zones which in general means: his penis, testicles and anus. Arousal for a man is like a stress release pill and he wants it even more when he is in a bad emotional state.

His arousal is easily created by two factors:

- The image of a naked female body and especially images of the female genitals.
- The touching of his genitals.

Getting older, a man will not become sexually aroused as easily nor be able to easily maintain the arousal. He cannot be happy experiencing the sexual act without strong excitation. His physiological capacity to feel sexual energy has substantial limitations. His body by nature is a very poor sensual instrument. Touching the different parts of his body does not give him much pleasure and does not excite his sexual energy unless he develops his sensuality. Unfortunately many men hardly develop their sensuality at all. Poor sexual education, watching pornography and having had negative sexual experiences in the past due to sexual failures close the door for the man to enter the rich world of a creative and loving sexuality. Most men never discover the art of eroticism and sensuality. They can reach orgasm easily but this will not make them sexually happy.

So a man constantly suffers from his male instinct which literally drives him crazy. When he is very young he has a constant erection and ejaculates quickly. When he gets older he can not get an erection as easily but needs to feel it, and again when he gets it he ejaculates and loses it. Having a partner does not stop him from constantly dreaming about having sex with other women. Because his sexual arousal is based on the two factors mentioned above it fades in a long term relationship and he needs new stimulation. This can be a new woman. Seeing her body is an exciting image for him. But not even this can save him from his various complexes and he feels compelled to treat the woman and her body in ways she does not deserve. Most men are deeply rooted in the belief that they have to do everything in bed and that the main pleasure of sex is the pleasure of orgasm, which they have to provide for themselves and for their female partners. Many men complain about women being passive in bed. However, deep down every man likes to proclaim himself 'the master' of his woman's body. He likes to feel that the woman belongs to him, that only he can enter her body and that she is devoted to him.

One can feel sorry for the predicament men are in.

The good thing is that in sexuality a man is like a child. Or even like a good faithful dog. He does not need much. If he is given a little more than he expected he is eternally grateful and eternally happy. Just like a child. From my experience working with men for many years I can paint a very clear picture of what happens to a man in terms of sexuality here in England, the country where I live. Maybe in other countries it is different, though I've had clients from other countries and it seems to me that everywhere the situation is similar. I will try to summarise my observations. Men in England are completely disorientated about sex. Their minds are poisoned by pornographic images, from having a lot of sex and masturbating from an early age. They have sex uncontrollably and with many partners until they get married. They are very influenced by the propaganda telling them that they need a large penis. They think that the more they ejaculate the better. It is in this way they experience their manhood. I think men in all countries have the same way of experiencing their sexuality. Most men in the world have depleted their life energy and sexual potential by the age of forty. This is confirmed by the statistics on Viagra consumption. These days a lot of men start using Viagra in their early thirties. In England more and more young men are turning to doctors having problems with impotence and premature ejaculation. More and more men in their thirties experience depression, anxiety and chronic fatigue. More and more men are using tranquillisers and drugs to cope with modern life and their own psyche. Less and less men marry and have children before being in their forties. More and more men prefer to remain single and have short-time relationships with women. Moreover, large numbers of men prefer to engage in unnatural forms of sexuality, such as sadomasochism, orgies and other sexual games. One night stands have become a common phenomenon these days, not only for single men but married ones as well. The market for prostitution in England is enormous and even with the addition of a lot of women from Eastern Europe and Asia all these millions of women definitely have a successful business. All because a man needs to feel like a man, which means he needs to express his reproductive function. A man needs to experience, often just to check and be reassured, that he can be aroused and ejaculate. The factual experience of this arousal and ejaculation is included in his basic characteristics as a man. He goes to the football game, he talks about politics and he gets aroused and ejaculates. This is what it means to be called a man. If his reproductive function fails he panics. And this panic is what has brought me most of my clients, not the desire to become good lovers for their women. This is understandable. As I have mentioned above, men do not need much. If they have sex from time to time they are happy and have no complaints. The woman is the one who needs much in order to be sexually happy. Still the question remains: Is a man truly happy simply because his reproductive function is confirmed? I don't think he is. The fact is, he has little choice.

In England most women decide to engage in a long-term relationship when they are around thirty or older. In many countries (in Russia and Eastern Europe) women get married at twenty-two or twenty-three. Though this does not make any difference. In every country the reason why women get married, sadly enough, is not because of their desire to create a happy sex life with their husbands. If you ask the women: "Why are you getting married?" most of them will probably answer: "I want to have a family, a home and children." They obviously want to live together with their men in one place, but having sex is not a woman's priority. But for men, having sex with their wives is their priority. It is the main reason why men get married. They believe that they will be able to satisfy their male instinct regularly and that only this way will they be happy. Women are of course aware that sex should be present in their lives as a couple. Yet usually they do not pay much attention to this side of their relationship. In England for example men and women usually live together for several years before they announce their engagement. About a year later they get married. By that time their sexual passion has faded a long time ago. Most couples have sex once or twice a month as the bodies call for sex. Their bonding and connection is based not on physical love, but on the many other elements of getting used to each other. They share interests, friends, relatives, housing and children. Many couples would call this love and do not realise that the lack of physical love is like mould beginning to develop. This mould can suddenly grow and destroy everything that has been so carefully built. Usually the man is the one who suffers when the sex life is almost absent in a marriage. His instinct does not disappear. A man watches pornography and masturbates or visits prostitutes. A man cannot live without experiencing physical closeness to a female body. I would like to repeat this again: not having sex is unbearable for a man. Women can live without sex for months and they naively believe that men can do the same. Couples usually do not talk about their feelings around sex. Eventually a man finds a way to satisfy his sexual needs on the side of his relationship. In England men prefer not to change partners because they can't see how having a different woman would make a difference to their sex lives. I have heard from many men these words: "A wife should be a good friend and a good mother. It is better to have sex on the side. It's easier." This is what they say but I don't think they truly believe in it. Every man desires to have a regular sex life with his life partner. Unfortunately, women often don't want to understand this. When a man is sexually hungry he cannot commit to anything including his work. It is hard enough for a man to cope with his own body and even harder to also find a way to satisfy his woman. A woman usually expects the man to satisfy her sexual needs without doing anything to help him. The man's body is rarely shown much loving attention by the woman.

The truth is, the male body is sensitive and needs the same care and love as the female body. For centuries there is rooted in peoples minds the stereotype of men being strong and tough. This takes away from them the opportunity to open up and develop their ability to be sensual and erotic. Men's clumsiness, haste, and sometimes rudeness is not their fault, neither is it their sexual nature. Yes, a man might ejaculate quickly but this does not hurt the woman. What hurts the woman is his inability to caress her body with gentleness and care. Slow and gentle physical touch does not become a habit to men due to a lack of opportunity to develop such touch, to 'rehearse' it. Girls and young women are often engaged in gentle caresses with mothers, sisters, brothers, fathers, friends...and, of course later with their children. Even adult women are hugging and touching each other with tenderness. Boys cease to experience gentle embraces often from the age of five or six. "You are a man!" they are told and are then firmly patted on the shoulder when they cry. Grown men pat their girlfriends on the shoulder and later their wives. Most men are unaware that this patting is frustrating instead of arousing to a woman and that it kills her desire to make love. Only a woman can help the man to become an affectionate and gentle lover and to become more erotic and sensual. When she knows how to lead her man during lovemaking she will help him become a man that will treasure her body and touch her in the way she wants to be touched. But she needs to touch him first. Only a woman can help the man be able to enrich their sex life with beauty and poetic touches. If she initiates everything they do: kissing, hugging, stroking, she will invite her man to participate in the most significant event of his life – the school of lovemaking. He cannot be the teacher of lovemaking. Only she can. Woman can lead man towards opening himself up into being a completely new kind of lover; subtle, relaxed in the body and deeply connected to her and her world of feelings. The man will be nothing but grateful to a woman that teaches him this. In this sense he is like a child.

Men's And Women's Bodies Differ But
Their Senses Are The Same

The idea that male and female bodies are sexually very different is widely spread. The idea that women need less sex than men is also widely spread. Women do need sex but of a different kind than most men can provide.

Women usually do not pay much attention to the question of how to understand the male body. They do not worry too much about how to satisfy their men sexually; it seems straightforward. They worry more about how to attract men and then about how to keep them from being attracted to other women. This is the main reason why, especially in long term relationships, women have sex with their men which with time starts to feel like a duty.

Men on the other hand always worry about how to satisfy women sexually. They are looking for all possible information on female arousal, mostly referring to stimulation of the female genitals and erogenous zones.

But finding the G-spot or other 'hot spots', knowing how to 'give pleasure' orally, how to stimulate the anus, knowing many sexual positions or even learning about different kinds of orgasms and becoming skilled in providing them often is not enough to feel emotionally connected to your partner through touch.

Male and female bodies are different in how they relate to their sexual instincts. When a couple share love and when they care about each other their bodies are similar in many ways. Both men and women have the same physical and emotional reactions to loving and caring touches, to eye contact that reflects mutual attraction and adoration, to a soft gentle voice, to words of love and to the smell of the loved one. When both physical bodies become the transmitters and reflectors of a feeling of love men and women experience no difference in their physical bodies. The lovers become as one body.

This sense of oneness happens because our human senses are the same. We can feel similarly about a particular image, taste, smell, texture or sound. We can all say about a picture: "I like it". We can like the same song, food, or sensation from touching a fabric. It is the same with physical love. There are a lot of touches and romantic elements in lovemaking that men and women can enjoy and appreciate in a similar way. The purpose of physical love is to create these romantic elements and touches to make a man and a woman feel as if they were one physical body.

Sexual Diet

The same way the physical body needs the right food, it also needs the right sexual diet. Any diet has the purpose of improving health and establishing a sense of well-being. Any diet answers the questions: what, when and how much? Your body needs the same questions answered regarding the sexual diet. We all need to know what kind of sex to have, when to engage in it and how much sex is good for us to stay happy and healthy sexual beings. We also need to help our partners become these happy sexual beings.

So, what are the answers to the three questions?

1. **What kind of sex to have?**
2. **When to have sex?**
3. **How much sex to have?**

I differentiate between four types of sex to help you maintain and organise your lovemaking better in any period of your life.

Four Types Of Sex

Through many years of professional practice and through personal experience I have distinguished four types of sex. These definitions are here to help you in the understanding of how couples can express physical love every day, any time they want to.

You have to consider three things in deciding what is best for you and when:

- **Correctly estimate your physical state in the moment.**
- **Look after your sexual energy during sex.**
- **Create touch that is loving and caring.**

My four definitions of four types of sex are not a dogma. They are meant to be an aid to establish the right time and energy for lovemaking. Bringing an understanding of these four types of sex into your sexual life will completely eliminate sexual hunger, sexual frustration and all sexual problems from your sex life. Your body will function sexually in a healthy and strong way, even though differently from what you are used to.

The four types of sex are:

- **Home sex.**
- **Celebration sex.**
- **Healing sex.**
- **Energising sex.**

Home Sex

Most men and women are working equally hard and often come home tired having no energy for passionate orgasmic sex.

Home sex is like being at home. The main purpose of home sex is to maintain the sense of closeness and to build up deeper intimacy and understanding between the partners. Our partner's body in home sex is a place where we can relax and feel comfortable. Any activity between two bodies is meant to relieve stress and create a sense of security and devotion. During home sex partners can even discuss problems and it will support their mutual care and understanding.

When men and women think about sex in this way, the body of their partner means everything to them; it is the best place in the whole entire world. Every day their affection will grow. As health food provides the right balance of nutrition for the body, home sex provides healthy nutrition for love to grow.

Home sex involves slow and gentle intercourse where both partners maintain a level of arousal that does not create a desire to strive for orgasm. They give each other hugs, gentle kisses and soft, easy massages. They can use romantic elements like listening to music together or slow dancing. The partners are focused on feelings of warmth and affection.

This practice allows 'sex' every day because the intimacy is similar to that of a hug. As there is no intention to create high arousal and orgasm the partners are learning about each other's bodies steadily.

Our body is changing every day as it is effected by our every day emotions. Home sex allows us to notice these changes and helps us restore the energy lost during a day of work. Home sex can last for any length of time. It is like taking a bath: you can stay in the water for five minutes or for one hour. These techniques can help couples that may not have been intimate for a long time.

Celebration Sex

This type of sex means a special day for a couple. Any couple needs special days to highlight their romantic feelings towards each other. Romantic feelings can easily fade because of our busy daily life. Celebration sex gives a boost to our sense of romance, as well as a boost to achieve high orgasmic states.

This practice requires preparation, planning and creativity. The purpose of celebration sex is to leave in our memory a special image and a special feeling. Celebration sex is a treasure which is kept in the heart to come back to when things are getting difficult or going wrong. It helps to restore positive energy. It is like a romantic film the couple can watch together to once again see the beauty of their partner.

The scenario for such a day can be simple and still include things we don't do every day: special music, food, lighting, clothes, rituals or a special environment. Whatever is planned it should not be difficult to do. It should be fun.

Elements of celebration sex are: erotic dancing, massages, romantic play and intercourse that brings the sexual energy up and down in waves eventually leading to a very high wave. Celebration sex includes incredible orgasmic states and very powerful orgasms through the whole body. These orgasms can be achieved through learning special techniques for cultivating sexual energy, directing it through the body and through developing the art of synchronisation.

Healing Sex

Sex is a powerful medicine. The techniques for healing sex are intended to release tension in body and mind, heal emotional wounds, help to eliminate stress and bring positive energy when something dramatic has happened. When a partner is ill or has a low level of energy the techniques for healing sex can help restore the body's energy.

Healing sex is very important in situations where a partner in a relationship is seriously ill, for example he or she has cancer or some kind of disability. Elements of this type of sex are: loving massage of different parts of the body, including giving attention to our partner's genitals. Loving touch awakens the flow of sexual energy. Then the partners can proceed to very slow intercourse in an appropriate position or to oral and manual techniques to stimulate arousal.

There are a wide variety of Healing Sex techniques that can make an ill partner feel happy and that can bring hope into his or her life when used in combination with feelings of love and care. The partner-healer should learn how to cultivate the right positive energy and radiate it towards his or her partner's body. There are many ways to achieve this that a lot of couples I work with might never have considered or have long since forgotten.

Healing Sex helps to bring physical love into the lives of people with a variety of physiological problems, diseases and disabilities as well as to people of older age groups. Using Unimacy's practical tools everyone can bring the joy of physical love to his or her partner.

Energising Sex

Energising sex is sex that activates our life energy. The best time for this type of sex is in the morning or afternoon. The aim is to wake up in our bodies extra reserves of energy for creativity and activity. Energising sex is a relatively short engagement in sexual activity, sometimes less than ten minutes. With special techniques the partners enjoy intercourse without any foreplay and without achieving very high arousal which means there will be no negative feelings afterwards.

Here, sexual arousal is distributed throughout the body and is sent to the brain in order to activate it. Energising sex is a boost or warm up, so there is not any loss of energy. Energising sex is especially effective before an important meeting. This type of sexual practice creates within the person the power, confidence and desire to win. This type of sex as well as the others requires from the partners great care and an ability to synchronise. And in this case to synchronise quickly, to channel sexual energy correctly in unison within a short period of time. For this type of sex a woman needs to develop the ability to make her vagina relaxed and aroused by using special techniques.

Touch Is The Main Language Of Physical Love

The sense of touch is our most fundamental sense. It is present in our lives at any given time. We relate to ourselves and to others through touch from the first minute we are born. We generally use our sense of touch naturally and unconsciously the same way we use our other senses (sight, hearing, smell and taste) unless we are out of balance.

A couple when in love constantly touch each other's bodies. A lack of touch creates a feeling of disconnection and doubt in our partner's love. But there are different kinds of touch. There is pleasant touch and unpleasant, even painful touch. Unpleasant touch creates negative emotions like irritability and anger. A pleasant touch brings a sense of trust and gratitude and a desire to respond in the same way towards our partner. This is why it is so important to develop the right touch.

Physical love requires that you develop the way you touch. It is like a language telling your partner about your love for them. It can create romantic feelings as well as bring sexual energy to life. A chain of romantic touches maintains this flow of love and sexual arousal. Contact with different parts of our body (hands, lips, hair, skin, genitals...) are equally important for the expression of physical love. A chain of romantic touches is richer if the whole body is involved in the touching. The skill lies in our learning how to do this and when.

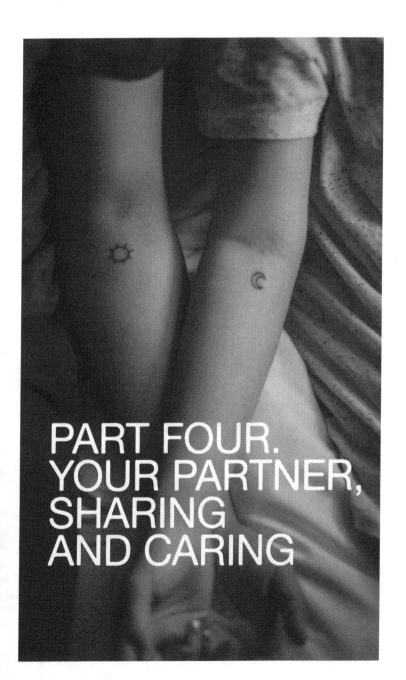

PART FOUR.
YOUR PARTNER,
SHARING
AND CARING

You Cannot Be A Good Lover For Everyone

The biggest step towards sexual happiness is taken when a man or woman knows his or her own sexual body well. When she or he knows what makes the body feel happy and healthy, what is good for it and how it likes to be touched in order to feel loved and nourished.

To be able to take care of ourselves better we have to be careful when it comes to engaging in sexual contact with people that follow mainstream ideas about sex. Their habits and tastes can put us into a state of confusion, stress, distraction and self-doubt.

It is difficult to completely avoid these people because most people follow mainstream ideas about sex. The concept of physical love as presented in the Unimacy system is new to our way of thinking and to our way of experiencing sexuality. Most people are not ready to adopt the Unimacy point of view straight away. The generally engrained habit of achieving physiological orgasm is considered a great and exciting part in the early stages of any relationship. This does not give much room for the possibly life-long lovers to start the practice of Unimacy.

However, you can gradually introduce your partner to Unimacy using a few simple elements of the system. You can start gently choosing something that is easy for your partner to enjoy. The main thing is not to give up or get frustrated with your partner who is still seeing things with different eyes. That would be like getting frustrated with a smoker who wants to give up smoking but still cannot.

By nature we are all 'sexoholics'. We need to be patient and loving when we want our partner to change his or her attitude and habits. Moving forward little by little every day is possible. Touching in new ways and noticing all the changes it brings to your relationship will create a constant loving emotional environment. Everything will work better day by day when you have an understanding of the Unimacy principles and a knowledge of the practices that suit your particular stage of life. Bodies change slowly but they do change. Exchanging new kinds of touch will change the body on a chemical level. The Unimacy techniques can change your mood, desires, feelings and habits. And learning new habits will renew any existing relationship as well as open you up to new possibilities if single.

Too Embarrassed To Start

Physical love becomes a creative process naturally and effortlessly if both partners are attentive and expressive towards each other using all of their senses. The partners smell each other's smell and enjoy it as though inhaling a wonderful perfume. Partners kiss each other's skin, lips or other parts of the body and the taste of the partner's body bring them great pleasure. They express this pleasure through sounds or words. The sound of the loved one's voice is also a pleasure. They look into each other's eyes and observe each other's bodies with adoration and joy. Their faces light up with love when they are physically close.

The truth is, the wonderful journey described above might never start even when both partners desire to practice conscious sex. Even when you and your partner agree with all the Unimacy ideas you may still experience a great awkwardness when trying to put into action what my system presents.

The only way to overcome this initial embarrassment is to start practising what I teach in my programs. With practice one becomes more comfortable with learning new ways of being and expressing oneself.

The Unimacy programs for couples are a great start. Any of them can be the beginning of a very beautiful journey for you and your partner towards each other and a happier future. It is even better if both partners do the self-exploration program at the same time.

Thereafter you can visit my website **www.unimacy. com** from time to time. This will allow you to introduce new elements of romantic love in you sex life at your own pace. Here you will continuously find new ideas on how to express your love physically in your sexual practice.

Remember, a conscious attitude towards sex is not automatically programmed in the human mind and body. Nobody is programmed to be a great pianist even if he or she eventually becomes a amazing musician. It all comes with practice. The first stage performance is the most difficult step for every musician. Then with time it can turn into an enormous pleasure and you will be living your dream life!

There is always the risk of your body, or the body of your partner, sabotaging the touches, movements and different elements of the Unimacy system thereby threatening your happiness.

The only way to get closer to where you want to be is TO DO IT. The Unimacy programs give you the gentle encouragement necessary to take the next step in the right direction.

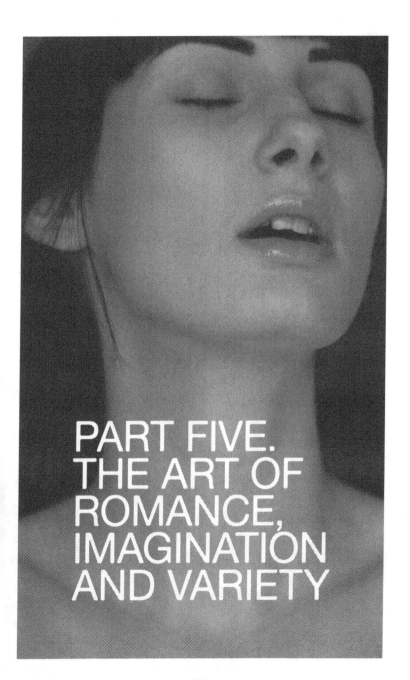

PART FIVE.
THE ART OF
ROMANCE,
IMAGINATION
AND VARIETY

The Sense Of Romance

Our imagination works with what is stored in our mind; everything we have ever seen, heard, tried and understood during our life. All these experiences form our desires.

These days most of us feel that the sense of traditional romance and beauty is lost. We do no longer see it in our lives, not even in art. Forty years ago in the sixties and seventies men and women still experienced the wonderful air of romance through films, music, fashion and visual arts. Today everything we see conveys a message of tragedy. Many films show violence or destruction. Contemporary art, music and fashion create in us a sense of power, freedom, energy and equality - but not romance.

It is really true that the sense of romance is missing from our lives at the present, but the elevated poetic feeling that in the past inspired all great people is still an important element of human life. Romance is the experience of melting into another, the experience of adoration and pure beauty... It is clear that years of going through the same routine of stimulating each other's bodies towards orgasm does not create romance.

Is it possible to feel like Romeo and Juliet throughout our whole lives? Maybe if Romeo and Juliet hadn't died but instead got married they would have ended up like many other dull couples. They probably would have argued and maybe ended up having an affair! I am sure that without being introduced to conscious sex their relationship would most likely finish the way it does for so many couples: with an, even though different, nevertheless tragic ending.

Conscious sex is an art, constantly created by two partners together. If the couple cease to continually create it they will regress and fall back into their old habits. The old desire for constant novelty, instant gratification and self-seeking will creep back into their minds and destroy their relationship. The desire for novelty and instant pleasure pushes men and women to search for quick ways to achieve arousal. This could mean having a new sex partner, using sexual stimulants or doing other things that distract from what truly brings lasting happiness.

How To Maintain Romance

There are three things that are important to maintain a happy sex life in a long term relationship:

1. To lay the right foundations for the sexual relations as soon as possible.
2. To monitor the development of the sexual relationship towards love.
3. To try to avoid causing unpleasant physical sensations during any act of intimacy.

Sexual relations is the most difficult area of human life and the most delicate and painful subject for many couples. Men and women need to learn the art of creating physical love. This involves using all of our senses within the context of the four types of sex as outlined earlier in this book.

Music

Music is a powerful source feeding our emotional resources. Filmmakers and advertisers know very well how to create romantic emotions in their audience. Without the special 'love-story' music in the background most love scenes would not resonate in people's hearts in a romantic way.

Music makes our body move and our heart beat. It can bring us to tears or laughter. If we use music during lovemaking we can tremendously change our focus and our ability to concentrate on the here and now. Music can take our thoughts away from every day events, problems and worries. It can diminish the importance of these events and instead highlight the feeling of love we feel towards our partner. It can synchronise us with our partner's emotions and energy and with the movements of their body.

What kind of music is best?

It is obvious that if we want to relax and take time to experience the slow flow of sensual touches we need to choose relaxing music. New-age music is considered relaxing, however most new-age groups use a very strong rhythmic background sound and fail to create romantic feelings. Instead they stimulate the brain and excite the body into rhythmically powerful movements leading to orgasm. Music for relaxation, yoga and meditation doesn't create any sense of romance either.

It is difficult to find the right music for lovemaking. Best is to choose songs or musical pieces that resonate with your heart as being 'love-story' music. You have to make your own compilations. Actively choosing the music that resonates with you will not only be an effort to prepare for your physical love practice but will also definitely make you think about your partner.

About whether he or she will like this particular music. Whether he or she will be inspired to hug, kiss, caress or dance to this music. Whether he or she will feel more romantic towards you.

By putting in effort and time in choosing the right music for the different types of sex, you are showing care towards your partner. This will allow you to get away from the routine and prevent you from taking your partner for granted.

Lighting

The room where you are going to make love should have special lighting. It doesn't need to be expensive or fancy. It can simply be a small pretty lamp that provides gentle light, preferably yellow or red. Yellow and red light make faces and bodies look glowing. The reflection of yellow or red light on the skin brings out a sense of smoothness and warmth. Men and women do not realise how much this small element can influence their feelings towards their partners.

Clothes

The beauty of a natural naked body is difficult to over emphasise. Some people are embarrassed to be naked in front of their partners. If you feel this way you can wear something, but the clothes should not be intended to have a seductive effect. It could be a T-shirt or simply a shirt. Find something to wear that makes you feel innocent, comfortable and easily open to skin-to-skin contact.

Food

Food is a wonderful element in lovemaking. Feeding each other mouth to mouth is a beautifully nourishing act. It opens up all our five senses in a deeper way. We can see the food and the mouth of our partner. We can feel, taste and smell. We can touch and we can make and hear the wonderful sounds of eating, kissing, laughing, talking while feeding each other.

Including food in lovemaking can create a beautiful sense of playfulness. When we touch the food and put it into the mouth of our lover, when we eat the food out of his or her mouth or hands, when we look at the lips of our partner and watch their movements we absorb the experience of our loved one bit by bit with a sense of adoration. Feeding each other with something delicious, light and appropriate to bring into the bedroom eases our tension and helps to create a cheerful atmosphere. We turn into teenagers.

Events

When we watch films, listen to music, walk the streets, spend time in nature or visit exhibitions we absorb into our soul the creative emotional energy of other people (artists, gardeners, architects). This energy helps us feel emotions for our partner.

Through events we share experiences and by visiting new places we can see our loved one with different eyes and see all the more clearly how wonderful they are. Through the artistic work of others we can develop our imagination when it comes to how to express our love towards our partner. We can also express our physical love while doing these things. We can listen to a song together and hug each other. We can walk hand in hand through the exhibition hall and feel the warmth of our partner's hand. We can watch a movie while holding a hand on our partner's knee. Physical contact while doing something together empowers our physical love.

If we already are in a passionate state of mind, touching each other while doing something together can bring out the passion even more. If we have been living together for a long time and the passion is gone, touching each other while we are out someplace warms us up. It creates more gentle feelings and a desire to unite in loving intimacy. The same thing happens when we hold hands, softly, gently and calmly.

Presents

Surprises light the fire of love. Little surprises are a wonderful expression of physical love. Giving something as simple as an apple, a pen, a CD or even a cup of tea to a long term partner is a big thing. In long term relationships everything works differently from how it works when a man and a woman are dating.

When we are dating little surprises often are not even noticed as the couple is carried away by the overwhelming feeling of sexual attraction. This is their main focus. In a long term relationship if a couple does not continue to surprise each other, even with little things like offering a cup of tea, it will seem as if they don't care any more. In the early stages of a relationship passion and sex colour everything. When people are together for longer periods of time the elements of care, small acts of love like offering a cup of tea and the warm hearted kiss that follows this offering, mean a lot. Giving a present is transmitting our loving energy through the gift. This is why these gifts will be treasured even more as they are manifestations of the effort and thought that have been put into them.

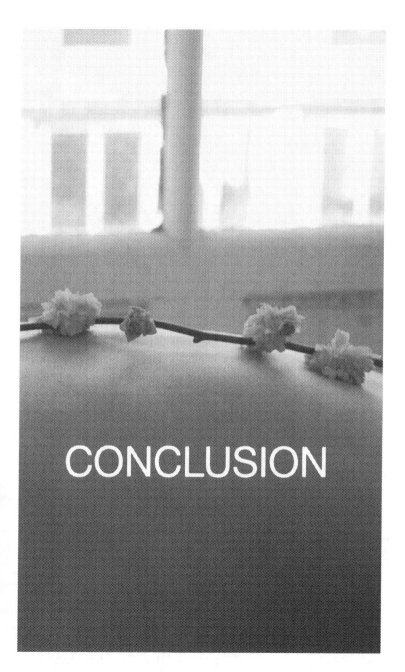

CONCLUSION

Physical love differs from just serving our basic sexual instinct. By learning about and loving your own body and by loving and learning about the body of your partner you extend your range of physical tools for expressing feelings of love. This will add to the longevity of your relationship. Physical love and Unimacy – enhancing union and intimacy - develop romance and maintain in both partners the sexual attraction towards the other.

The practice of Unimacy can tremendously enrich the sensual life of a couple no matter their age, sexual orientation or life circumstances. The knowledge is clear and the practice is simple and proven. The system has already changed the lives of many couples and single people that I have worked with over time.

Every child will grow into a man or a woman. It is important for parents to find a way to teach their children a conscious attitude towards sex. To protect them from the chaotic and thoughtless sexual behaviour inherent in today's youth, also strongly supported by various sources on the internet. Adolescents are at risk. Only parents can help them understand how to become sexually happy men and women. And first of all they have to be happy within themselves.

Taking time to learn more about this new approach to love and lovemaking will open you up to many forms of expressing physical love and counterbalance the unhealthy trends arising in our culture generally. It will give you a better understanding of your partner and deepen the physical and emotional connection between the two of you whatever the world throws at you. Unimacy can be practised by all cultures and age groups and is potentially the healthiest way forward for all of us wanting to enjoy sex and intimacy for as long as we still breathe!

I wish everyone the best for their relationship. Welcome to my practical programs. You will find them on my website: **www.unimacy.com**.

Lara Anderson

Printed in the United States
By Bookmasters